KW-299-969

Teenage
DIABETES

What it is and how you can get the best out of life

JUDITH NORTH

THORSONS PUBLISHING GROUP

Published in collaboration with
The British Diabetic Association
10 Queen Anne Street, London W1M 0BD

First published 1990

Copyright © British Diabetic Association 1990

*All rights reserved. No part of this book may be reproduced or
utilized in any form or by any means, electronic or mechanical,
including photocopying, recording or by any information
storage and retrieval system, without permission in writing
from the Publisher.*

British Library Cataloguing in Publication Data

North, Judith
Teenage diabetes: what it is and how you can get the
best out of life.
1. Young persons. Diabetes. Personal adjustment
I. Title   II. British Diabetic Association
362.1'96462

ISBN 0-7225-1884-6

Cartoons by Willow
Illustrations by Vince Driver

*Published by Thorsons Publishers Limited,
Wellingborough, Northamptonshire NN8 2RQ, England*

Typeset by Harper Phototypesetters Limited,
Northampton, England
Printed in Great Britain by Mackays of Chatham, Kent

1 3 5 7 9 10 8 6 4 2

Teenage DIABETES

Other titles available from Thorsons:
DIABETES HANDBOOK
DIABETIC COOKING FOR ONE
DIABETIC DESSERTS
DIABETIC ENTERTAINING
DIABETIC'S MICROWAVE COOKBOOK

Contents

Introduction

What? MORE words about diabetes?

Yes, but this book has the advantage of being written just for teenagers with diabetes. It isn't written for your parents or for the clinic staff (though you might find all sorts of other people sneaking a look at it). This book is for teenagers new to diabetes and for people with diabetes new to being a teenager.

The teenage years are a special time when you start to sort out who you are and what you want to be. There are many changes involved in growing up and at times your lifestyle may be in conflict with your diabetes. By the way, there is no such person as a 'perfect diabetic'. Actually, there is no such person as a perfect human being either; everybody is different. As a young person with diabetes you are only different in that you have one extra thing to consider that your friends may not have. So this book will give you information about diabetes, but it sees you as a teenager first, who just happens to have diabetes.

In case you are tempted to put this book down, having decided it will be another adult telling you what to do who doesn't understand about living with diabetes — don't! I have had diabetes since I was 8½ so I come under the heading of someone who has 'been there, done that, and bought the T-shirt'. Which doesn't mean I know all the answers, but hopefully the information here will help you to make your own decisions about your own life and how you want to fit diabetes into it.

Don't feel you have to read the whole book all at once from cover to cover. Use the Contents page and the Index to pick out the parts that interest you now. Some of it may seem obvious, or irrelevant to you, because teenage covers such a huge range of experience: it's up to you to pick out the appropriate sections. If you think I've left out something important, by all means write to me, care of Thorsons, and let me know.

A little history

Diabetes has been known as a condition for many centuries. The first English description of diabetes is from Thomas Willis in 1679 who wrote of 'the pissing evil' and describes the urine as being 'wonderfully sweet'. (Presumably he tasted it?!) The word diabetes comes from the Greek word for fountain or siphon — which well describes the frequent urination (passing water) and massive thirst you may have experienced before being diagnosed. Its full name is diabetes mellitus. Mellitus comes from the Greek word for honey; your urine would also have been very sweet.

A remedy for diabetes is mentioned in the Eherys Papyrus, written in Egypt in 1500 BC, 'a medicine to drive away the passing of too much urine'. The recipe included bones, wheat grains, lead, earth, and water — which can't have been very effective.

A major breakthrough in knowledge about diabetes came in Germany in 1889 when it was found that removing the pancreas from a dog led to it developing signs of diabetes. This showed that something in the pancreas is missing in people with diabetes.

This 'something' was discovered and extracted by Banting and Best in Canada in 1921, and named insulin. Before 1921, developing diabetes meant starvation and death in a fairly short period of time. The discovery of insulin brought a dramatic improvement in treatment (previously the only treatment was an almost starvation diet — thrice-boiled cabbage at least three times a week!) and life expectancy, but not, of course, a cure.

If you want to read more about diabetes in the early part of the twentieth century, *The Discovery of Insulin* by Michael Bliss (Faber, 1988) makes interesting reading. (It will make you glad you were born when you were, too.)

Section A

Newly Diagnosed?

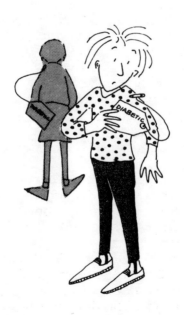

Chapter 1

What is Diabetes?

Diabetes is a disorder which develops when a person does not produce enough of the hormone (i.e. chemical messenger) insulin. Insulin works in all parts of the body and helps the sugar we get from our food to move from our bloodstream into our cells to give us energy. Insulin is released from the pancreas gland. The pancreas weighs about 60g and is found behind your stomach. Much of the pancreas produces digestive juices and throughout it are little 'islets' which contain the cells which make insulin (see Fig 1).

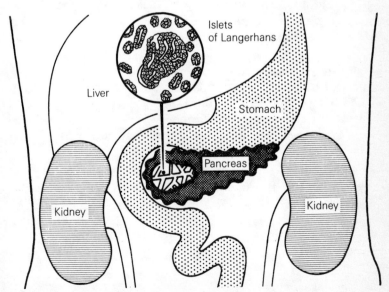

Fig 1 The pancreas, with inset showing the detailed structure of the insulin-producing cells, the islets of Langerhans.

In your case, these insulin-producing cells have been destroyed. Without insulin, the level of sugar (glucose) in your blood starts to rise.

Where does blood sugar come from?

Sugar in the blood comes from the food we eat:
sweet foods: sugar, jam, drinks (fruit and fizzy ones), etc.
starchy foods: bread, potatoes, cereals, flour, etc.
Fig 2 shows what happens to food after you have eaten a meal.

What happens without insulin?

Without insulin, your body is unable to convert the sugar in the food you have eaten into energy, or to store the sugar, so your blood sugar rises — particularly after meals. The kidneys can prevent sugar from passing into the urine, but when there is too little insulin, the blood sugar will reach the 'renal threshold' (renal means 'of the kidney') when sugar starts to spill over into the urine. (See Fig 3.) This gives rise to the three most common symptoms of uncontrolled diabetes. You may yourself have experienced these:

● **Passing a lot of urine**
In order to 'dilute' the excess sugar in your blood, water is taken from other cells in your body so more water needs to be passed out from your kidneys. You may have needed frequent trips to the loo, during both day and night.

● **Thirst**
Because so much water is leaving your body, you get a dry mouth and feel thirsty. You may have drunk litres of extra liquid — more than 20 litres (35 pints) a day is not unusual. Of course, this is made a lot worse if you choose to drink sweet fizzy drinks that contain a lot of sugar!

● **Genital soreness**
All that sugar in your urine may lead to soreness and itching around the end of your penis (if you're male) and your vagina

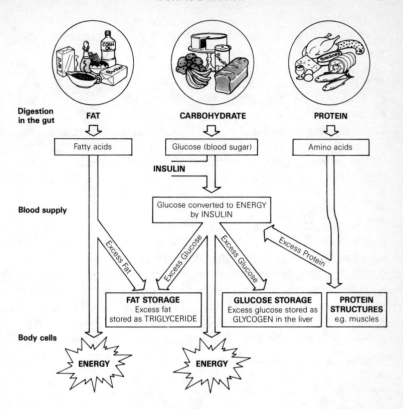

Fig 2 Normal metabolism: in the presence of insulin, glucose can be coverted to energy.

(if you're female). You may develop a fungal infection called thrush. This fungus thrives on sugar and gives you the itching and soreness. Both men and women get thrush. It can be treated successfully with special creams but, of course, it will keep coming back if you keep passing sugary urine.

What does your body do to create energy?

Without insulin, your body can't get energy from the food you eat. To keep surviving, your body must get energy from elsewhere, so it will start to break down your fat and muscle. Look at Fig 4 on page 17 and compare it with Fig 2. Getting energy from body fat and muscle may result in:

● **Weight loss**

This breakdown of your body fat to give you energy means you will weigh less.

● **Tiredness and weakness**

Muscle cells are also broken down to give glucose and then energy. This too will lead you to lose weight. In all the urine you are passing, you will be losing salts (that means chemicals like sodium chloride — which you know as table salt). Loss of body salts gives you muscular weakness and maybe muscular cramps.

● **Increased appetite**

Since without insulin you can't effectively use the food you eat, your body feels it is starving. Some people then start to eat more, particularly craving sweet things in an attempt to get energy — but this will only make matters worse.

When fats are broken down in the body, chemicals called ketones are produced. Nail varnish remover contains acetone which is a ketone. If you have a lot of ketones in your blood, people may be able to smell acetone on your breath. If a lot

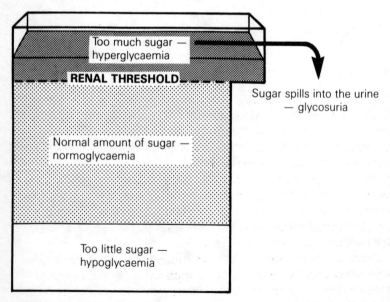

Fig 3 When the blood sugar reaches the 'renal threshold', it spills over into the urine.

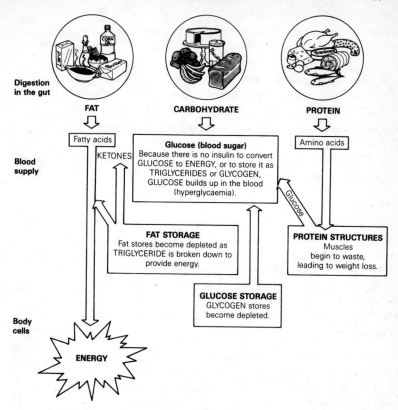

Fig 4 Breakdown of the body's energy stores.

of your fat is broken down, ketones build up in your blood. This is very harmful; think of it as 'blood poisoning'. Ketones also pass into your urine. There are tests which will show that your urine has ketones by the colour change on a strip which you pass through a stream of urine.

By the way, ketones will be produced when people slim but not, however, in the quantities that may occur when you have not enough insulin in your body. The reason why crash diets are not recommended for anyone is that too many of these harmful ketones may be produced.

Severe lack of insulin over some time leads to a condition called ketoacidosis, which has symptoms of increased urination, thirst, stomach pain, nausea, vomiting, weakness, confusion, tiredness (lethargy), and shortness of breath. This can make you very ill.

Along with the ketones, acids build up in your blood (more chemicals; vinegar is an acid, so is lemon juice; too much of them is unpleasant isn't it?). Your body tries to correct this build-up by deep breathing to blow off the acid gas. The deep breathing leads to drowsiness and then to a diabetic coma (which means a deep sleep, but you will need medical help to wake up). Prior to insulin being available, this was always fatal. Sometimes diabetes is not diagnosed until ketoacidosis develops. If that happened to you, you would be rushed to hospital as an emergency. Nowadays, with blood and urine sugar tests that are quick and easy to carry out, hopefully a doctor will do these tests for diabetes before such a crisis is reached. However, if your diagnosis was delayed, don't blame your family doctor. With only one person in 300 under the age of 16 developing diabetes, s/he may not have seen many cases before.

We'll return to ketoacidosis later. You need to know how to avoid it, preferably, and how you must get medical help if it does develop.

Types of diabetes

The type of diabetes you have is insulin dependent diabetes. This usually develops between birth and the age of 30. You produce little or no insulin and have to inject insulin to survive.

Non-insulin dependent diabetes (sometimes called Type II diabetes, whereas yours is Type I diabetes) usually develops over the age of 30. People with Type II diabetes produce some insulin but it may not be enough or it may not work properly. These people may control their blood sugar levels by a careful diet or a combination of diet and tablets. These tablets are not insulin, but substances which get a person's own insulin supply moving when it is needed. Insulin may be required later if the tablets do not lower the blood sugar enough. People with Type II diabetes do not go into a diabetic coma if they stop taking their tablets, but their diet may be much more restricted than yours — so don't assume they have an easier time of it.

You won't be able to change to tablets as you get older: they only work if you have your own insulin also available. Some women develop diabetes when they are pregnant (gestational diabetes), which may or may not go away after the baby has been born. None of the other types of diabetes ever go away.

There is one new case of diabetes diagnosed every 10 minutes in the United Kingdom; 250,000 have insulin dependent diabetes and probably about 40,000 of these are under the age of 20. These numbers are all guestimates since no one has ever registered all of us and counted us up; about three times as many people have non-insulin dependent diabetes. There are an estimated 30 million people with diabetes diagnosed worldwide; 20–25 per cent of these people are insulin dependent. Overall, that is 1–2 per cent of the population. So, there are a lot of us about!

Chapter 2

Diagnosis

What are they doing?

It is possible that you had not been feeling well for quite a while before diabetes was diagnosed — you may have had more colds, for instance, or developed boils, or just generally not had much energy. Research is showing that it may take months or even years for diabetes to develop to the point where you experience some of the symptoms mentioned in Chapter 1.

If you had these symptoms severely, you may have been taken to your local hospital and admitted for a while. If you and your family were worried about your health, perhaps you went to see your family doctor (general practitioner) who tested your urine or blood for sugar and then referred you to the hospital.

Most family doctors won't have much experience of youngsters with Type I diabetes. It doesn't mean you are more ill because you are sent to a hospital, but there will be more expertise you can learn from there. Perhaps later you could talk to your family doctor and pass on some of your knowledge, which will help others in your position later.

Facilities for people with diabetes vary depending on where in the country you live. Some places now have special diabetes centres which may be separate from the rest of the hospital. In other hospitals you will be seen at an out-patient clinic. If this clinic is a children's clinic (it depends how old a teenager you are), you may find that other conditions are being seen, not just diabetes.

If you are older, you may be seen in an adult diabetic clinic, which can be a bit like a cattle market. They may be full of frail, elderly people and you may get depressed. You may have a long wait and little time to say how you feel. Most people, including the medical staff, don't now think these clinics are very helpful. So, if you do find yourself in a clinic like this, instead of getting fed up, spend the waiting time thinking about how it could be changed to be more 'user friendly' and try making suggestions to the staff.

Places also vary in whether they admit you to hospital when you are newly diagnosed with diabetes. If you are in ketoacidosis, however, you will be admitted because you will urgently need replacement of the water your body has lost. This will be done by putting a needle into one of your veins and dripping in water and salts. You will be given insulin too. If you are not that ill, you will still need to start to take insulin — which you may do as either an 'in' or an 'out' patient.

There can be good things about being admitted to hospital. As an in-patient you get 'looked after' and you can learn about diabetes in a concentrated way. However, as you may be a bit shocked and scared, you may not be able to take in much of what you are told — and you may become swamped and more unsure. But you may be able to meet others with diabetes and learn together, and share some of how diabetes feels.

The hospital routine won't be how you will live at home so there will be many adjustments to be made to your insulin dose over this initial period. Before diabetes was diagnosed, your food and exercise levels may have changed so there will be some 'trial and error' to find what is an appropriate system for you. Please don't think that if your insulin dose is increased you have 'got worse'. Ask other people: doses vary a lot. Sometimes, too, you may have a few remaining insulin-producing cells having a 'final fling' — this is called a 'honeymoon' period, and, as you might guess, it doesn't last!

If you are admitted to hospital, it will give your family a chance to adjust to diabetes without adding their worries to yours. However, barriers and misunderstandings can build up if everybody doesn't talk together. Everybody will feel sad at times, too; there is a feeling of loss. Sharing the sadness and crying will help — bottling up all your feelings inside makes them larger; maybe they get twisted, and this doesn't help anyone enjoy their life.

Who are 'they'?

Newly diagnosed with diabetes, you will meet a group of people who have useful knowledge and training. Your doctor may be a paediatrician (children's doctor) with an interest in diabetes. Don't be offended if you are an older teenager and see a paediatrician, since some paediatricians see people until they are over 20! If you are older, however, you may see a physician who looks after adults with diabetes.

If your physician specializes only in diabetes, s/he may be

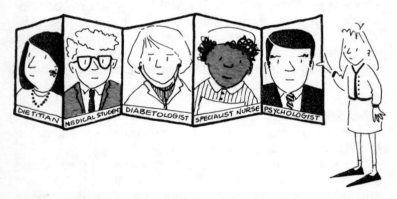

called a diabetologist. If your physician sees people with other conditions affecting glands in the body (the thyroid gland for instance — some people lack the thyroid hormone), s/he may be called an endocrinologist. (The system of glands in your body that give out hormones into your blood is called the endocrine system.) If your doctor is a general physician, that means s/he has specialized in medical conditions, not surgical ones.

The 'chief' doctor will be the consultant, who, once appointed, will usually stay at the same hospital until retirement. The next level down is the senior registrar who will stay in one hospital for several years. Then there are qualified doctors who are learning about different specialties — you won't get to know them very well as they move on within a year. If your hospital is attached to a medical school, you may meet medical students too.

Your doctors have had a long training, care about helping people and have taken an oath not to gossip. As with everybody you meet, you will like some of them better than others. They are human beings, not gods, remember, so do try to be open and honest with them about how you feel about diabetes and how you manage your treatment.

Most health areas now have diabetes specialist nurses, whose job it is to help you with the day to day management of your diabetes. Most of them are women, but more men are now going into nursing so hopefully this will be changing. These nurses don't spend all their time in the hospital. They may visit you at home and they may visit your school to give your teachers information about diabetes.

The hospital team will include a dietitian, who knows all about food. The dietitian may also specialize in diabetes and/or children. You may also meet a psychologist who can help you to talk about your feelings and any difficulties you may have on a personal level. You are likely to see a chiropodist sometimes, who will be interested in helping you to take care of your feet. The importance of this will be explained in Chapter 7.

Now you have diabetes, your medical team will be part of your life. You will get on with some of them better than others, but that is OK. Remember they are likely to have useful information that will help you to live your life to the full. Only very rarely are they ogres! Unless they also have diabetes (and don't forget, they may well have), they won't totally know how to live with diabetes. Learning about diabetes from other people is different from learning about diabetes from your personal experience. Everybody is different, so part of living with diabetes is to become your own medical expert. Don't think you have to learn everything at once, though, or you will get so you can't see the wood for the trees.

There's more about diabetic clinics in Chapter 12.

Chapter 3

What You Do to Treat Your Diabetes

Insulin — how does it work?

Diabetic or not, whenever we eat, our blood sugar rises. If you don't have diabetes, food is the signal to your pancreas to pour out insulin. During the half hour after eating a meal, insulin levels in the body rise. As insulin moves round the bloodstream, it allows sugar (glucose) to enter the cells of the body. About two hours after a meal, both insulin and blood sugar levels fall back to the fasting (that means non-eating) level (see Fig 5).

Insulin levels keep closely in step with blood sugar levels throughout the day and night. Between meals there is a steady background release of insulin to match a background level of sugar which is supplied by your liver. This sugar supplies enough energy to keep your cells 'ticking over'.

Since you have diabetes, you are no longer producing insulin. You need to give your body this background level of insulin, plus extra boosts of insulin to help digest the food you eat at mealtimes.

Unfortunately, insulin is a protein-like substance so it cannot be taken by mouth. Proteins, that is things like meat and eggs, are broken down into different substances by stomach juices. If you did swallow insulin, it would be destroyed by the stomach before it could be of any use in digesting your food. Therefore, insulin has to be injected.

Before you do your first injection, you may be very scared of injections. Probably the only injections you've ever had before were at the dentist, or vaccinations. After you've done the first one, you will know that insulin injections are quite different from the other sorts. It wouldn't be true to say they never, ever, hurt, but most of them don't. As you are only injecting under the skin, any pain is soon gone too. (This is a bit heavy — but remember, you will die without injections of this stuff.)

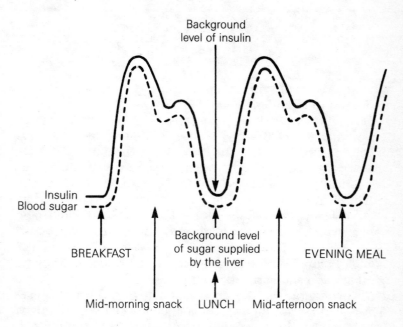

Fig 5 Insulin levels keep closely in step with sugar levels throughout the day.

Your medical team (probably the nurse) will teach you how and where to give injections. It is not a good idea to wipe your skin with an alcohol wipe to clean it, since this will toughen your skin and make injections more difficult in the long term. You may feel a bit clumsy, slow and nervous at first. With practice, it really will get as easy as cleaning your teeth.

It is important for people you live with to have a go at injections, both on themselves (*without* the insulin!) and on you in case you ever need help — you might break an arm. However, if you rely on someone else injecting you fre-

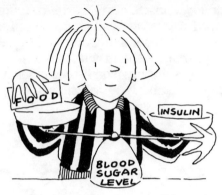

quently, you will severely limit your life and activities. It is more fun to be independent, isn't it?

If you find your skin is very sensitive sometimes, you can try putting an ice-cube on the spot before you inject. Try this if you want, but you will find the insulin may be absorbed less quickly — and you do need to be somewhere that has ice-cubes!

The insulin you inject will take time to get to the same part of your body which contains the food you have eaten. The rate at which insulin is absorbed varies for several reasons. You can use this fact creatively. If you know your blood sugar is high before you inject, you can lower it more quickly by getting the insulin absorbed more quickly.

The injection site you choose affects the absorption rate. The rate is fastest from the stomach, followed by arms, thighs and buttocks. However, activity plays a part. If you've been cycling, insulin injected in your thigh will move round faster.

Heat also increases the rate of absorption. This means hot air temperature, a hot bath or shower, or rubbing or warming the spot after your injection.

Often the site you choose may be just the one you find most convenient to get at with the clothes you are wearing!

It is *very* important to vary your injection sites, and not to keep injecting in the same place just because you think a new spot might hurt. Your tissues will get damaged and insulin will not be absorbed efficiently if you keep using the same spot — and you may develop unsightly lumps and bumps which will take a long time to go.

It is wise to wait a few seconds (count up to ten) before withdrawing the needle after an injection. If a little insulin still leaks out after this, though, don't worry, you won't have lost much. You may see a little blood if you touch a small blood vessel with the needle, which may give you a bruise later. Again, this is not something to worry about.

A very few people are allergic to some of the preservatives used in insulin solutions (it is not often an allergy to the insulin itself). If this happens — you might get a rash or a sore spot — see your doctor. There are many different insulins on the market so you can always change brands.

Types of insulin

Different types of insulin work for different lengths of time. You may have guessed by now that to get a balance between your injected insulin and your blood sugar level, you will need a boost of short-acting insulin to cover meals, plus a long-acting, background insulin. There are many ways of achieving this balance. The aim is to avoid wide swings in your blood sugar levels, so that you will feel well now and in the future. Balancing insulin and blood sugar levels depends on several things:

- the type of insulin you inject
- the time of day you inject your insulin
- the times when you eat your meals
- the amount of food you eat
- the type of food you eat
- the frequency, timing and quantity of exercise you take
- the way you feel emotionally
- the weather.

This may look dreadfully complicated, but you don't get all of them at the same time. You need to learn your own patterns. There isn't one insulin which is 'best'. It is a matter of which insulin best suits *you* at this time in your life. There are no rules which say you must have one type rather than another. This is something to talk over with your doctor to find a system which fits in with your lifestyle.

Briefly, at present there are two main types of insulin, clear and cloudy, though there are about 40 varieties of these two on the market. Clear insulin is quick-acting and cloudy insulin is slow-acting — but the dose you give and the other factors

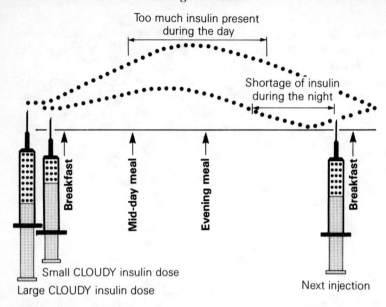

Fig 6a If the single, daily dose of cloudy insulin is too large, there will be too much insulin present during the day; if it is too small, there will be a shortage of insulin during the night.

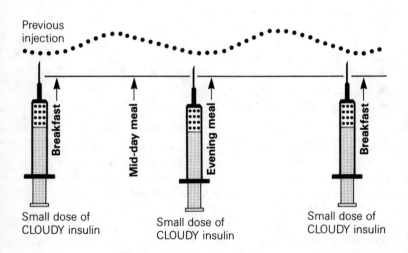

Fig 6b Smaller doses of cloudy insulin are shorter-acting than a single, daily dose.

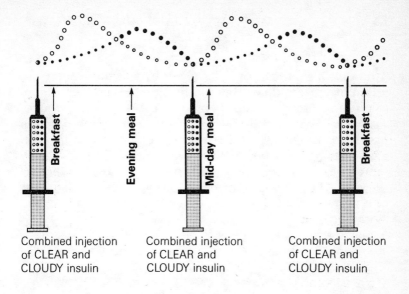

Fig 6c A combination of clear and cloudy insulins ensures peak as well as background levels of insulin.

---

listed on page 27 also affect the action of different insulins. There are these overall comments which are true:

● if your blood sugar is consistently high, you need more insulin
● if your blood sugar is consistently low, you need less insulin
● bigger doses of either type of insulin last longer
● a large dose of clear insulin may last nearly as long as a small dose of cloudy insulin.

Figs 6a, 6b and 6c illustrate this.

Options for injection systems range from one daily injection of cloudy insulin (very inflexible — you'd be stuck with fixed meal times) to an injection of clear, short-acting insulin before each meal, with one injection of long-acting, cloudy insulin every 24 hours (very flexible, but more injections). Whatever system you use, make sure you know how long 'your' insulin(s) work, and when their action is at its peak — this is the key to fitting diabetes into your life. There's more about food and timing later on (Chapter 4).

Devices

Although insulin can only be given by injection, there are different ways of doing this. Plastic syringes and needles are free on prescription to people with insulin dependent diabetes. They come in 50 and 100 unit sizes and different packaging. You may prefer a rigid plastic case to a plastic 'bag'. The markings may be blue, brown or black. The barrel may be round or square. The needle covers vary as does the feel of the needles. Try out as many as you can and see which suits you best — though you may find your local chemist won't stock them all, which may restrict you a bit.

Glass syringes are still available but they are heavy, need sterilizing and are bulky to carry around — not

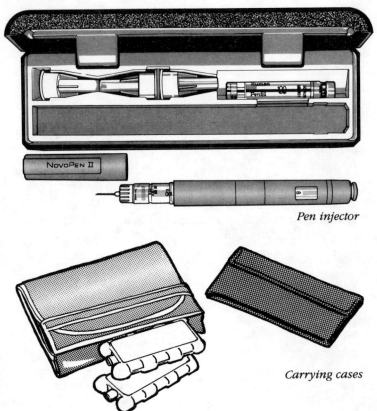

Pen injector

Carrying cases

recommended. There are various 'pen' injection devices on the market. These carry a cartridge of insulin inside that removes the need for carrying bottles of insulin and syringes separately and look very discreet. These are recommended as they are very portable and user friendly.

Some people choose to have their insulin delivered from a pump. This means having a needle under your skin at all times which has a thin tube attached to it, connected to a small box containing insulin and a pump. You set the rate to give a background level of insulin and increase this at mealtimes. The needle must be moved every few days. The pump has to be removed when swimming or bathing and you need access at all times to medical help in case the mechanism goes wrong. However, you can keep a level blood sugar with this system and it suits some people very well.

There are also 'jet' injectors available which squirt a high-pressure jet of insulin under the skin. They are very expensive, cumbersome and not painless. There is a worry that the high pressure may cause damage to body tissues if they are used for a long time. Again, they may suit some people.

If pumps had been invented first, syringes (particularly pen devices) would have been greeted as a breakthrough, and a vast improvement. Yes, other people can be funny about needles and syringes, but try to see that as their problem and don't make it yours.

As you will have gathered by now, insulin is only one part of the system of living with diabetes. You need to know about food as well. The next chapter fills you in.

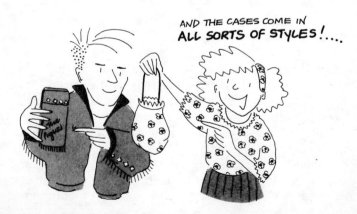

AND THE CASES COME IN **ALL SORTS OF STYLES!**....

Chapter 4

Food

Those of us with diabetes need to learn to be aware of what we eat and when we eat it. Compare yourself to a car: now you are injecting the insulin your body needs, you are on manual transmission instead of automatic. As with cars, this is not always a disadvantage.

Many people still believe that a 'diabetic diet' is very restricted and unappetizing. This is NOT true — the recommended food plan for people with diabetes is no longer a 'special' diet. It is the same healthy eating scheme recommended for the general population. The only difference with diabetes is that you have to take a closer look at the amount you eat and balance it with your insulin intake and exercise. You also have to think about timing your food intake.

The basics

Food is made up of three main components — carbohydrates, proteins, and fats. To have a balanced, healthy diet, everyone needs to eat all of these. Foods may contain mixtures of all three, two of them, or just one. Think about what might be in milk, eggs, pastry, cheese, bananas, and cabbage. Check your answer with somebody if you are not sure.

Carbohydrate is found in two types of food:

1. Starchy foods e.g. cereals, pastries, flour, potatoes, fruit, milk.

These foods have to be digested before they turn into sugar in your blood. High-fibre (that is 'brown') varieties of these foods, and also fruit, vegetables and pulses are recommended

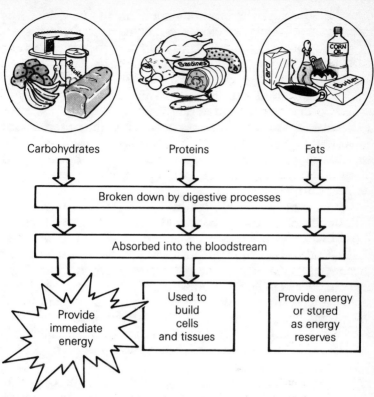

Fig 7 The three basic components of food.

for everyone. (Pulses are the seeds of one family of plants. You will meet them as things like kidney beans, lentils, chick peas, and the beans in baked beans.)

Fibre is the plant part of foods that can't be digested (broken down) into other things that will feed your body. In that case, why should we eat it? Food without fibre in it can be digested with less effort. This means the muscles in your digestive system may become lazy — which may lead to constipation, gall bladder problems and bowel disease, none of which are comfortable to have.

For those with diabetes, the presence of fibre slows down digestion and thus the rate of sugar production and absorption. This helps to even out your blood sugar levels and so avoids extreme swings. The slower production of sugar from the food you eat also gives the insulin you have injected more time to move from your injection site to where it is needed in your gut to help store this sugar.

By the way, since the fibre in food absorbs water in your stomach, you may need to drink more when your food is higher in fibre.

2. Sugary foods e.g. honey, instant sugary desserts, jam, sweets, soft drinks (the non-diet variety).

Because these foods do not contain any fibre, they do not need much digestion and their sugar passes rapidly into the bloodstream. This causes a rapid and large rise in your blood sugar. This increase may not last long, so you may be swinging about again.

After reading about carbohydrates you might be wondering, if you stopped eating carbohydrates altogether, would you then not have to inject insulin?

Please don't try this. Without carbohydrate in your food, you would not be well-nourished, which is not good for growth or overall health. You would always feel hungry. Also, if there are no foods taken into your body that contain sugar, your body just starts to produce sugar from its reserves. This means you will lose weight (which might be what you want) but the poisonous ketones will build up in your blood which will make you very unwell indeed.

Protein provides the building materials for the cells and tissues of your body. It is found in meat, fish, eggs, dairy products, cereals, and some vegetables. Meat and fish do not contain any carbohydrate unless this is added during the cooking. For example, a steak has no carbohydrate, but steak pie has carbohydrate in the pastry. Animal proteins may also contain fat. Things like milk contain carbohydrate, protein and fat; cheese contains protein and fat.

Vegetable proteins usually contain carbohydrate and/or fat as well. For example, the pulses and cereals contain protein and carbohydrate.

Fat is required in your diet both to provide energy and to be stored as energy reserves. However, people actually need very little fat in their diets. All food is measured in calories, but fat is higher in calories than other types of food. (Calories are a way of measuring the energy-producing value of food.) Calories 'in' need to equal calories 'out' — if you eat more calories than you use up as energy, the calories will be stored as fat and you will put on weight.

Designing your food plan

The aim of your food plan is to have a 'balanced diet'. That means you are eating enough food so that you are not hungry, and that the food contains carbohydrate, protein and fat so that your body is growing healthily. Your food intake should also keep your weight steady at whatever level is appropriate for your height, build and sex. You have probably noticed in shops various pots of vitamins and minerals, and may have read advertisements in magazines encouraging you to add these to your diet to make you more healthy. If your food has the correct balance of carbohydrate, protein and fats, the vitamins and minerals you need will be automatically included, so there should be no need to take any vitamin and/or mineral supplements.

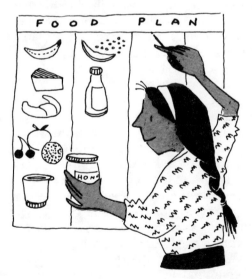

With diabetes, you need to find the balance that evens out your blood sugars and satisfies your hunger. You also have to sort out which foods will satisfy the sudden energy requirements which happen when you do strenuous work or sport, and what foods work for you when you need to treat a low blood sugar. This is something which will be covered in detail in Chapter 9.

To sort out your food intake, there are several factors to take into account. This is where your dietitian can give you a lot of help too. You need to consider:

● What is your total food requirement per day?
● What do you enjoy eating?
● When will you want to eat?
● When will you need to eat?
● What are the best foods to eat?
● Which foods can you try to eat less of?

No foods are 'forbidden'. Many people believe that 'diabetics can't eat sugar' so you may find yourself explaining about food and insulin to others at times.

Exchanges

For convenience, in the UK, we talk of foods that contain 10g of carbohydrate. The 10g are also sometimes known as exchanges, portions or lines. 'Exchanges' can be used as a name for the system because a 10g portion of, say, fruit at lunch can be 'exchanged' for a 10g portion of bread, if you feel like it. Be careful about this. The total weight of an apple is likely to be much more than 10g, but much of it is water: it contains only 10g of carbohydrate. Depending on the food, the amount of it containing 10g of carbohydrate will differ. 'Lines' is a term not much used now — on that system you had to keep a balance of red and black lines from a diet sheet. (A diet sheet is a list of foods with their carbohydrate, protein and fat contents or values — not a piece of material that you can eat!) As a very rough guide to start from (again, you need to find out how *your* body works) 2 units of short-acting insulin will balance 10g of carbohydrate.

In America, people with diabetes may also count the number of grams of fat and protein in their meals, so they use fat and protein exchanges too. This makes for quite a complicated system. You may also hear people talk of 'free' foods. In the UK, these are foods that contain no carbohydrate and so can be eaten 'freely', which means as much of them as you fancy. Foods like meat and cheese used to come under the heading of free but now people are aware that a lot of fat isn't good for anybody, free foods would be things like lettuce and cabbage — so this isn't a very useful way to talk of foods.

Lists of 10g carbohydrate exchanges are available from your dietitian and from the British Diabetic Association. You will learn to develop an 'eye' to estimate how many grams there are in unfamiliar foods. Please don't imagine that you will need to carry weighing scales with you everywhere (it is only the *carbohydrate* weight you need so the total weight won't help) or that you need to be accurate to the decimal place. If it says on a packet of crisps that it contains 12g of carbohydrate, you count that as one exchange.

Food labelling is becoming much more detailed now, so reading the labels in the supermarket or the cupboard is a good way to learn about food and what it contains. The ingredient listed first on a label is the one the product contains most of. So if sugar is a long way down the list, there isn't much there. Beware of the 'No added sugar' claim — glucose, dextrose, honey and other 'sugars' may be added. This doesn't mean you can't eat these things, but think about it when you do so.

Diabetic products

You may have noticed that there are 'diabetic products' around in some shops. They are usually sweet foods in which the sugar has been replaced by another sweetener which doesn't contain ordinary table sugar. These products are not necessary for anyone with diabetes. Many of them contain a lot of sorbitol, which may give you diarrhoea. They are very expensive too and may be high in calories — so don't think they will help if you want to slim.

On the other hand, sugar-free diet drinks are useful and now are readily available. If you find an eating place that doesn't have them, it is worth asking for them and maybe even writing to the management to encourage them to buy some in the future.

If you like to sweeten tea or coffee, some of the artificial tablet sweeteners will have a place. Saccharin used to be the only one available. You can still get this but many people don't like the 'metallic' taste it has. 'Nutrasweet' is often seen on labels and can be bought as a powder to sweeten cereals, for instance. You can't, by the way, use this in cooking — so if you make custard, don't boil the nutrasweet up with the milk but add it afterwards. There are many different sweeteners on the market — try them and see which you prefer.

Chapter 10 has more information on food, including alcohol and eating out.

Chapter 5

How Am I Doing?

Having diabetes means you have to balance 'sugar in' to your body with 'sugar out'. This is something you control (or try to — it often isn't as easy to do as to say). If it doesn't produce its own insulin, your body can't do this for you — remember you are on 'manual' now, not 'automatic'. Blood sugar levels are affected by four main factors:

food
illness or other stress} RAISE your blood sugar level
insulin
exercise} LOWER your blood sugar level

You may not know what your blood sugar is by how you feel. As you get more used to having diabetes you may be able to guess your level quite well but it is easy to get it wrong by guessing.

When your blood sugar is low (this applies to everyone, not just people with diabetes), your body sends out adrenalin which is the substance that encourages your body to release the sugar it has stored in your liver. Adrenalin is also released if you are afraid, to help you to fight or run away by releasing sugar into your blood to give you more energy. When you are afraid, you often feel shaky. If your blood sugar is low, you may also feel shaky. You will need to check which is correct at the time. For example (and you don't need to actually try this out!), if you get in a fight, afterwards you are likely to feel very shaky and stressed — and have a high blood sugar.

So, how *do* you know what your blood sugar level is? What is the range of values you are aiming for?

Everybody's blood sugar varies. For people without

diabetes, the range of variation is quite narrow, but their blood sugar will also rise after meals and if they are stressed. The range to aim for, to keep your diabetes balanced, is between 4 and 10 millimols per litre (mmol/l). The units of measurement used in America are different — to translate, you multiply by 18. That is a range of 72 to 180 milligrams per decilitre (mg/dl).

The non-diabetic range is sometimes quoted as between 3.5 and 8 mmol/l, but it is probably wider than this since people who do a lot of sport, for instance, may experience low blood sugars around 2 mmol/l. Also, people under a lot of stress, say after a car accident, may show higher readings than 8 mmol/l. For you, keeping between 4 and 10 mmol/l is trying to stay within the 'normal' non-diabetic range. (Mmol may not mean much! If it helps you to see things, 4 mmol/l is the same as a quarter of a teaspoon of sugar in a litre of water.)

Years ago, testing blood sugar levels was very complicated and could only be done in a laboratory, so people with diabetes tested for sugar in their urine. (Remember that if your blood sugar is high, this sugar spills over into your urine.)

However, this test didn't give you much information since sugar doesn't usually spill into your urine until your blood sugar is above 10 mmol/l. Since the urine has been in your body for some time, the result will be an hour or two old as well. Also, it won't tell you if your blood sugar is too low; and the test is messy and inconvenient to do.

Blood tests

In the past ten years, it has become possible to test your blood sugar level at home by taking a small spot of blood from a finger (or toe or ear lobe if you prefer). You will be taught how to do this test by your diabetes care team, and they may want to check your technique from time to time. The change in colour on the test strip is a timed chemical reaction; you won't get an accurate answer if you are sloppy about timing it correctly or wiping the strip.

There are various types of testing strips available and devices for making a skin prick to extract some blood. These are both free on prescription. It is worth trying several of the skin prick devices if you can, until you find one with which

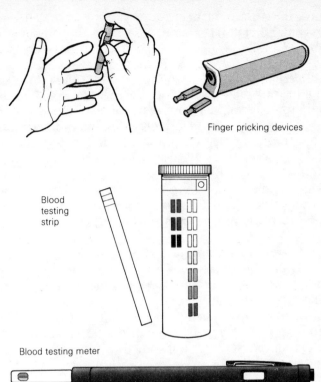

Finger pricking devices

Blood
testing
strip

Blood testing meter

you are comfortable. There are meters available which will give you a digital reading of your blood sugar level from a strip. These are quite expensive (not available free on prescription) and some are bulky if you intend carrying them around. They must also be handled with care and kept clean. Providing you can see the colour changes (it may be a problem if you are colour blind), you don't need a meter. However, some people prefer to have that accuracy — your choice.

A few tips:

- it is easier to get a spot of blood from warm fingers
- your thumb and forefinger are often more sensitive; try using the other ones
- sugar on your fingers will give you an incorrect reading, so will some hand creams — wash your hands first
- don't keep strips in the fridge — they are made to read accurately at room temperature

- you can re-use the lancet for pricking your finger until it gets blunt (but don't use your lancet to prick someone else's finger).

If a urine test shows that your urine does not contain sugar, you only know that your blood sugar was probably below 10 mmol/l up to a couple of hours previously. You won't know how far below 10 mmol/l it might be now. So blood tests are not only more simple to do anywhere and give an up-to-date blood sugar value, they will also tell you if you are close to too low a blood sugar. Blood sugars below 3 mmol/l are in the hypoglycaemic region (hypo = low, glycaemia = blood sugar). If you are 'hypo', you will not be functioning well and will need to eat some sugar quickly. Hypos are covered in detail in Chapter 9.

There are no hard and fast rules about how many blood tests you should do. To start with you may want to test several times a day to help you learn what changes your blood sugar and how you feel at different levels. Frequent testing will also help you to set up a system of insulin injections and food that fits in with your lifestyle. It will always be useful to increase the number of tests you do if something changes in your life — perhaps your job or exercise pattern, or if you travel further than going to school or work.

Your doctor may give you a book in which to write down your blood sugar test results. Sometimes you can be made to feel that this book will be judged like an exam and the doctor will pass or fail you. It doesn't have to be like that.

Writing test results down is useful when you are first diagnosed, to help you to sort out a system of insulin, food and exercise that works for you. After that it will be helpful:

- if you are ill
- if you are changing your lifestyle, e.g. a new job or sport
- if you are travelling
- if you change your number of injections or type of insulin
- if you change your food, e.g. become vegetarian
- if *you* feel you would like to know your blood sugar level.

It is important to do blood tests at different times of day sometimes, to get an overall picture of your balance. Once again, there is no such thing as a 'perfect' anything. Sometimes you will be fed up of the whole business of balance and not want to mess about with any tests. When this happens, do resist the temptation to make up the results in your book — this isn't of any value to you or to your diabetes care team. There are also various ways of fiddling the results, like leaving the blood on the strip for less time (you can work out for yourself what that will do to the result!). But, overall, who are you kidding?

It is also not very useful just to write down the test result without thinking a bit about it. The result you get may have an explanation which can be used to make adjustments to your insulin, food intake, exercise, etc. Don't jump to conclusions, though. If your blood sugar is high before lunch, for example, it could be:

- you've eaten too much during the morning
- you've had less exercise or physical work than usual
- worry or stress
- not enough insulin
- a faulty test carried out.

There are other explanations too, and sometimes there just doesn't seem to be any reason at all. Unless you are ill, don't change your insulin on the result of a single test, but only when you see a trend over, say, three days. The test, remember, shows how your previous injection worked, not what your next dose should be.

Before you make any adjustments, you must know how long your insulin(s) are effective and when they peak. Then there are various things you can do:

- change your insulin dose
- change your type of insulin(s) and/or the balance between them if you use two types
- change the timing of your injections
- change the amount of food you eat
- increase the number of your injections
- alter your injection sites
- alter your exercise pattern.

This long list still isn't complete. Stress will also affect your blood sugar, and ways of tackling this will be suggested later. You may also be affected by hot or cold weather, though not wet or dry, unless you get a lift when it is raining!

Everyone is different and so is everyone's diabetes. There is an amount of 'trial and error' in finding a balance. This may sound very complicated but you don't have to do it all by yourself. You can get help and ideas from the staff at your clinic and from other people with diabetes. One word of warning — if you do make changes, make them one at a time, then wait a day or two to see what happens before you try something else, if you think another change is necessary. As time goes on, your confidence will increase and you will get to be your own expert in your diabetes.

Are you feeling a bit overwhelmed? If so, don't panic — you don't have to take all this in at once.

Things you might like to try

Why not make a chart like this one and fill in your answers about how you felt/feel about being diagnosed with diabetes?

Key ideas	Then	Now?
Emotions	How did I feel?	
Fears & fantasies	What was the worst thing that was going to happen to me?	Did it?
Family/friends	Who helped? Who didn't? How did they react?	
Successes/frustrations	What went well/badly?	
Actions	What did I do? What did I not do? What did I stop doing? What did I avoid doing?	

Overall, life is better/worse, easier/harder because . . . ?
I can consider changing . . . ?
Assuming that you have yourself had diabetes for more than a week or two, if you met someone who had just been diagnosed, what pearls of wisdom would you like to share with them?

If you are very recently diagnosed, see if you can contact someone who has had diabetes for some time and ask them the question.

Chapter 6

Why Me?

Even though diabetes has been known as a condition for thousands of years, still no one can answer the question 'Why did I get diabetes?' The research on trying to answer this question fills volumes. We do now know some bits of the jigsaw, if not the whole picture. Part of the problem is that people only go to the doctor when they have already developed symptoms of diabetes. It seems that the development of diabetes certainly starts to take place many months, probably several years, before those symptoms that are recognized as diabetes show themselves.

Old wives' tales

You may hear several 'old wives' tales' about the causes of diabetes in general, and your diabetes in particular. They are almost certainly untrue, so don't accept them without asking someone else (preferably someone on your diabetes medical team) about them. It is NOT TRUE that Type I diabetes is caused by:

- eating too many sweets, junk food, or anything else connected with food and eating
- anything you have done, or not done
- anything members of your family have done, or not done
- the surroundings/area you live in.

You may say that having diabetes is bad luck, but it is not your fault or anybody else's.

Genetic factors

We do now know that people who develop Type I diabetes are born with an increased risk of developing it. Everyone's body is made up of cells. These cells contain genes, which are the materials that determine which characteristics you will have, e.g. your hair colour, height, etc. The genes you have come from genes your parents have, but they can be combined in different ways — which is why you are not the same as your brothers or sisters.

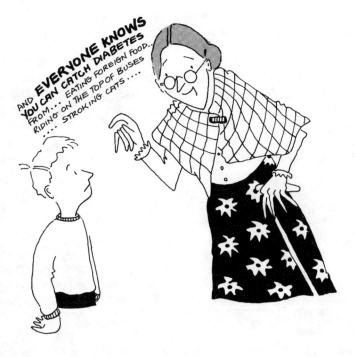

Most (98 per cent) of the people with insulin dependent (Type I) diabetes have a particular type of material in their genes, which is found in at least three different parts of their cell centres. So we now know which bits of genes are nearly always present in people with Type I diabetes. These bits of genes are the parts which help your body to recognize 'foreign' substances. Unfortunately, for some reason not yet known, your body has decided that your insulin-producing cells (these cells are called 'islet' cells after the way they are found in your pancreas) are 'foreign' so your body attacks and destroys these cells.

Though these genetic factors do play a part, they are not the whole story. About 30 per cent of the general population also carry these genetic markers, but they don't ever develop diabetes. Identical twins have exactly the same gene pattern since they are formed when a single fertilized egg splits into two — so they would both or neither carry the markers for diabetes. If they do carry these markers, still only half of them develop diabetes. So, in order to develop diabetes, something else needs to act as a 'trigger'.

The trigger

At the moment it seems that this trigger may be a virus. The word virus comes from the Greek word for poison. Viruses are *very* small and often cause disease, in people and plants. (Anything you were vaccinated against as a young child would be a viral disease, e.g. polio, measles, whooping cough.) In the case of diabetes, the virus would cause your body's defence system to start attacking your insulin-producing cells. At least, that is the theory.

This is no ordinary virus, however. It has yet to be identified and it appears that the 'infection' takes place a long time before diabetes symptoms develop, since the blood of newly diagnosed diabetics rarely shows any recent viral infection. However, the blood of many newly diagnosed people with Type I diabetes does show antibodies (these are substances which act against, or destroy cells) to insulin-producing cells.

This is an exciting line of research because it may, in the future, lead to vaccinating people with 'diabetic' genes to prevent them from developing diabetes. Fig 8 may make this a bit clearer.

There isn't a definite 'carrier' gene for diabetes, so even if one of your parents has diabetes, you can't say you have got it from them — though your risk of getting it will have increased. Stress is sometimes called a cause of diabetes, but this has not been proved. However, stress does cause disturbances to your body's disease-fighting system so it might make some people more likely to be affected by a virus infection. Don't forget that this has to be a stress that occurred probably years before you developed diabetes — so you can't blame any recent upheavals in your life.

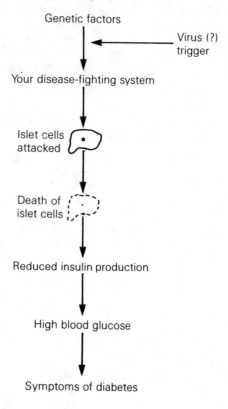

Fig 8 The cause of Type I diabetes?

If you have brothers or sisters, they might be interested to know that they have a 1 in 15 to a 1 in 30 chance of also developing diabetes. Remember, though, that doesn't tell you much since 'chance has no memory'. At the moment there is nothing they can do, or not do, to prevent this happening. It is possible to check whether they have the 'diabetic' genetic material, but it is a very expensive test. If they don't have this material, they won't get diabetes — but even if they do have these genes, they still may not get diabetes unless they meet the 'trigger'.

By the way, Type II diabetes does not seem to have this gene pattern and the types do not seem to be linked. So your diabetes is not related to your grandmother's, who perhaps developed it at age 60 and had to eat very carefully but didn't need insulin.

Cure?

As well as not knowing what causes diabetes, or how to prevent it, we also can't cure it — yet. For the moment you must assume you will have diabetes for the rest of your life. If you were ill before diabetes was diagnosed and since you have been taking insulin you feel fine, you might be tempted to think you don't need insulin any longer. If you decide to give up insulin injections to see what happens, you will find quite soon (within a day or two) that you will be ill again, and you may be carted off with the flashing blue light to hospital. Learning by experience is a good method, but just for once perhaps you could learn by *my* experience of the ambulance!

Do be wary of any newspaper or television reports that say a cure has been found for diabetes in some distant corner of the world. If this is true, it won't be a small comment, it will be headline news. Also, any new treatment isn't instantly available at your local hospital. Remember that though we all know that man has been to the moon, it is not yet the place for your summer holiday.

There is more about research and the future in Chapter 21.

Chapter 7

Fantasies, Fears and Feelings

You may have noticed that bad news gets more space in newspapers and on television than good news. You may find that some people delight in telling you bad news about diabetes. Do check out any information you are given with someone who is knowledgeable and up-to-date about diabetes. There are many myths (that is another word for fairy stories) you might hear. To answer some of them:

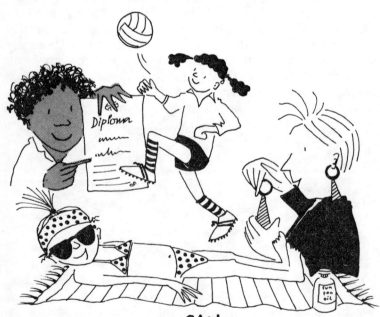

PEOPLE WITH DIABETES **CAN....**

- It is NOT TRUE that people with diabetes get gangrene in their feet by cutting their toe nails!
- It is NOT TRUE that you will go blind from wearing tight crash helmets or riding hats or from bumping your head!
- It is NOT TRUE that you must avoid football, swimming or any other sport!
- It is NOT TRUE that girls with diabetes have to go to hospital for their periods!
- It is NOT TRUE that girls with diabetes can't have babies or that boys with diabetes can't be fathers!
- It is NOT TRUE that diabetes makes you stupid!
- It is NOT TRUE that having diabetes makes you more likely to have any other physical or mental illness!
- It is NOT TRUE that people with diabetes can't have their ears pierced!
- It is NOT TRUE that people with diabetes can't sunbathe!

You may meet others. If you are worried, check them out.

General health

People with diabetes can have vaccinations and visit the dentist in the same way as anyone else. Yes, you can eat the sugar lump that may come with the polio vaccination! With the dentist, there is no reason not to have a local anaesthetic (that is the unpleasant injection that 'freezes' your gums) but if you need a general anaesthetic (that is the one that puts you to sleep) you should go to a hospital dental clinic. Try not to arrange appointments at a time of day when you might have a low blood sugar, though this probably won't be a problem if you are very nervous. You should tell the dentist that you have insulin dependent diabetes. If you visit an optician you should mention it too.

'Complications'

Have you heard about these? They may have been used as a threat: 'If you don't keep to your diet/keep your blood sugars normal, you'll get complications before you are very much older.' What does this really mean?

It is a fact that, as a group, people with diabetes (both Type I and Type II) are more likely to get certain types of physical problems later in life. 'Later' in your case will be after you have had diabetes for at least 20 years. It seems, though it is not proved yet, that if you avoid wide swings in your blood sugar levels over long periods of time you are less likely to develop these problems.

There are no guarantees, however, in anyone's life: '1 in something' estimates of risk don't tell you what will happen to *you*. It seems that 25 per cent of people with Type I diabetes don't get any of these problems. Perhaps they have another gene arrangement that 'protects' them? No one knows the reason for this yet. Please note that if you do develop one of these side-effects after 20 or more years of diabetes, it doesn't mean you will then go on soon to develop all the others — they don't necessarily occur together.

The 'good control' that is so often talked about doesn't mean being perfect — but it is sensible, isn't it, to aim to be as healthy as you can and feel well from day to day. It probably isn't healthy to be obsessional about control and let diabetes take over your life, though.

So what physical problems are we talking about?

Your heart
Your arteries (which carry blood from your heart to the rest of your body) may harden and narrow (arteriosclerosis). This may occur in many older people, particularly if they smoke, are overweight and take no exercise. People with diabetes seem to be more likely to have this happen. Severe arteriosclerosis is known as coronary thrombosis. This is when blood clots form in deep veins (which carry blood back to your heart) and arteries, and travel to your heart causing blockages — hence heart attacks and maybe death. Eating a low-fat diet, minimizing stress, and taking exercise will all help you to have a healthy heart. So will not smoking.

Your eyes
People with diabetes are prone to damage to the tiny blood vessels in the back of their eyes. This part of your eye is called your retina and the condition of damage is called retinopathy. If untreated, damage to your retina may reach a point where vision is lost and blindness may result. It is now possible to treat

such damage using a laser, providing it is found early enough. The laser produces bright pin-points of light which can be focused on your retina in the places where extra blood vessels have formed. The light burns a tiny spot to prevent these extra blood vessels from spreading and damaging your sight.

Damage to your retina in the early stages does not affect your eyesight, so you will not know if anything is developing. (If you *are* having difficulty seeing, you go to see an optician, just like anyone without diabetes.) So it is very important to have the backs of your eyes examined every year when you have had diabetes for five years or so.

The examination may involve having drops in your eyes to make your pupils (see Fig 9) wider so that the retina can be seen more easily. These drops can sting and you will not be able to drive for some hours afterwards. If the day is very sunny, you may find wearing sunglasses for a few hours will help. Some clinics now have cameras so that photographs can be taken of your retina (you may not need drops in your eyes for this — it depends on the make of the camera). The photographs can then be compared from year to year and any changes treated if necessary. So, get your eyes checked by an expert regularly — you can avoid losing your sight.

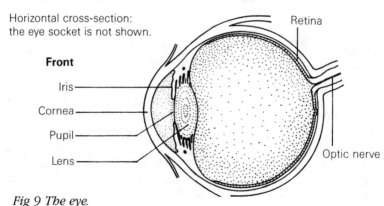

Horizontal cross-section: the eye socket is not shown.

Front

Iris

Cornea

Pupil

Lens

Retina

Optic nerve

Fig 9 The eye.

Clouding of the lens of the eye, cataracts, are also more common in people with diabetes, usually when you are older, say over 50. Improving your blood sugar and insulin balance may reverse this clouding. Cataracts can be removed by an operation. You would need to wear glasses or contact lenses to correct your vision afterwards.

Your extremities

Nerve damage (neuropathy) may occur with diabetes, most likely in your legs and feet. Early symptoms of this are 'pins and needles', numbness and pain. You can get these feelings for other reasons too, so don't panic every time you get cramp. Neuropathy will build up over some time; again it isn't inevitable and won't happen until you are *much* older.

Any loss of sensitivity to pain may result in unfelt injuries, particularly to your feet. If your blood sugars are consistently high, injuries don't heal quickly and may become infected. This may lead to ulcers and possibly gangrene. (Gangrene means body tissues have died. Amputation stops its spread from being fatal.)

Because of the possibility of such problems, it is important for you to take care of your feet. It isn't reasonable to say that because you have diabetes you should never go barefoot or that you must always wear 'sensible' shoes — but do be careful and try to follow these suggestions:

- Wash your feet every day in warm water and soap. Dry them well.
- Cut your toe nails straight across and not too short.
- Wear the right shoes for what you are doing whenever you can.
- Make sure your shoes fit properly.
- If you get a foot injury, see a state registered chiropodist, don't try to treat it yourself with a corn remedy, for instance; these can damage your skin.

Impotence: neuropathy combined with narrowing blood vessels may affect other 'extremities' — which is one way of describing a penis! There is a higher incidence of impotence from physical causes in men who have had diabetes for a very long time — not in teenagers. (In fact, impotence is not uncommon in older men, diabetic or not.) Very often the cause of impotence can be psychological (in your mind) and it may be temporary. If impotence should happen to you (again, we are talking about 20 years from now), do seek expert help. It doesn't mean the end of your sex life.

Your kidneys

Kidney disease is also more common in people who have had diabetes for a long time. One of the warning signs for kidney disease is showing protein in your urine, and this is something that will be checked at a clinic visit. It is important that you treat any urinary infection (cystitis, for instance: you will know you've got this if you feel a burning, 'nipping' sensation when you pass water) effectively so that it doesn't move on to your kidneys.

It seems that people with high blood pressure are more prone to kidney disease, so this is another thing to check as you get older, and to take medication for if necessary. Blood pressure is checked by putting a tight cuff round your upper arm and reading figures from the height a column of mercury is raised. Blood pressure is written as two figures, say 100/70. The top one goes up if you are stressed — motor racing drivers, just before the start of a race, have readings of over 200. The bottom one goes up if your blood has trouble getting through your blood vessels because they are narrowed. Thus, stress will raise your blood pressure, and so will worrying about complications.

These last few paragraphs explain what is meant by 'complications'. Please don't now go and feel depressed and 'I might as well do all the destructive things I can because life won't be worth living in a few years.' That isn't true — none of these things is inevitable. If you think about it for a second, none of us knows what is round the corner — do we?

Having diabetes brings out different feelings in different people, and you get different feelings at different times. If you feel sad, try not to bottle that up. Crying sometimes helps. There is nothing wrong with being sad, or with being angry — which is also something you might feel about diabetes. Some ways of expressing anger are more help than others. Kicking the cat or fighting your family isn't helpful — it isn't their fault.

If your anger gives you masses of energy, is there a way you could use that constructively? Do you want to shout? Try shouting into the wind on a walk. If you want to beat something up, hit a cushion or a ball. If it makes you brood, how about writing or drawing something? These may not be easy ways to express anger, but using them sometimes may be easier than screwing up relationships with other people.

By the way, hypos can also be called a 'complication' of

diabetes — they are not forgotten or ignored, they come in Chapter 9.

Section B

Day to Day Living

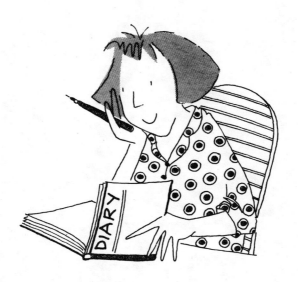

Chapter 8

More Insulin Information

In case you were wondering, insulin used to be extracted from the pancreases of pigs or cows. This was not identical to the insulin that human beings produced. Nowadays you are likely to use 'human' insulin that is identical in structure to the insulin produced by humans.

This human insulin is made in one of two ways. Either purified pig insulin is adjusted to get it to correspond exactly to the structure of human insulin, or bacteria are programmed to manufacture human insulin. Insulin is, in fact, the first product of genetic engineering to be marketed. Human insulin is *not* made from human pancreases. There is absolutely no risk of you contracting AIDS or any other disease from it.

Storage

Your stocks of insulin should be kept cool and dark. The salad part of a fridge is ideal. Don't put it in or near the freezer or ice-making part. The molecules (that means the smallest part of a substance to retain the properties of that substance) will be damaged if insulin is frozen — so if you are travelling by plane, keep your insulin with you; the baggage compartment gets very cold in flight.

On the other hand, insulin will also be damaged by boiling or getting very hot, so avoid leaving it in the glove compartment or boot of a car, or on the parcel shelf. If you are travelling to very hot or very cold places, it might be a good idea to keep your insulin in either an insulated bag or a small

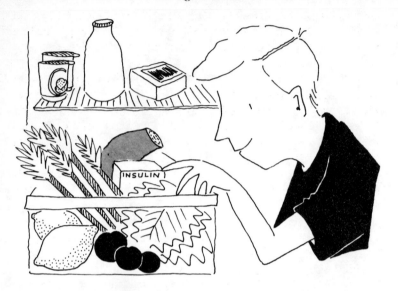

plastic insulated flask. It probably wouldn't ever occur to you to do this, but don't try to transfer your insulin to another type of bottle — a recipe for disaster.

If your insulin does get too hot or too cold and you have no other supplies, it is still safe to use it. However, if some of the molecules are damaged, it may not be as concentrated as it was and you may have to increase your dose to get the same effect. If your clear insulin goes cloudy, get a new bottle out and throw that one away.

It is perfectly all right to keep the bottles you are using out of the fridge. In fact, it is wise to keep your current bottles at room temperature as it can be painful to inject cold insulin.

If you use a pen injector it will come with a case. If you don't want to carry spare needles or insulin cartridges with you, you can keep the pen in a pocket or bag quite safely. For bottles and syringes, there are soft cases available (not free, though) that fit into pockets of bags, or hard cases that are useful if you are hiking, etc.

Injection worries

It is not generally necessary to clean the tops of insulin bottles before you draw up the insulin, or to clean your skin, since insulin contains preservatives and bactericides (they kill germs). Also, don't swab your skin with alcohol wipes as this will make your skin become like leather in time. Use soap and water if necessary.

If you have read many detective stories, you may be worried that if you inject air with your insulin, it may kill you. It takes a *lot* of air to do this and the air needs to go into a vein, so you need not worry. You are taught to get rid of air bubbles in your syringe before you inject so that you inject the correct dose, rather than some units of insulin and some of air.

There is also no danger of injecting into large blood vessels (veins or arteries) if you stick to the recommended sites. Any bleeding will only be from small (capillary) blood vessels and will soon stop. You may be left with a bruise if this happens, and insulin may circulate faster. Infected injection sites are *very* rare — the bactericides in the insulin solution help to prevent this.

Don't worry if a little insulin leaks out after you withdraw the needle (even if you have counted to ten before taking the needle out) — you will lose very little. If you want to try to avoid any leakage, you can pull the skin to one side before or after injecting to close off the puncture.

You will probably have realized that insulin will take time to move from your injection site to where your food is being digested. This is why you are usually recommended to inject yourself before you eat. How long before depends on what your blood sugar is at the time, and what you are going to eat. This is another pattern to sort out for your own body, and rigid set times don't usually work too well.

If your blood sugar is low before a meal, you should eat immediately after injecting or you may be hypo before you finish your meal, particularly if it is a high-fibre meal which will take time to digest to produce sugar in your blood. You can even inject after a meal if your blood sugar is very low — only it can be very easy to forget your injection altogether then, which isn't a good idea later on. If your blood sugar is high before a meal, you can safely wait longer than 20 minutes before eating. How long you can wait and what is 'high' in this case is likely to be different for different people.

Plastic insulin syringes are now available on prescription, which is free to you since people with diabetes (those on medication that is; not for Type II diabetes when on 'diet alone' treatment) are exempt from all prescription charges. You need to fill in a form from your family doctor and you will then receive a certificate which is valid for five years. You may be asked to show this certificate when you go to a chemist with a prescription.

Syringes can be used several times. You need to change them when the needle feels blunt or when the markings rub off. Also, if you get the needle dirty, by dropping the syringe perhaps, or bend the needle, maybe when replacing the cap, you would be wise to get a new syringe out. If you are going to use a syringe again, always store it with the needle cap replaced.

The next chapter goes into more detail about high and low blood sugars.

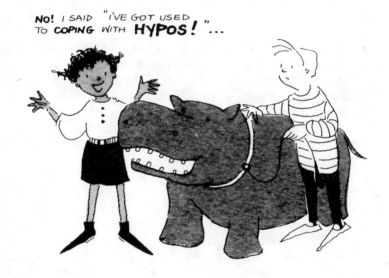

Chapter 9

Living with Hypos and Hypers

To go back a bit, 'hypo' (pronounced *high-po*) is short for hypoglycaemia, or low blood sugar. Scientifically, this is classified as when your blood sugar is below 2.2 mmol/l (40mg/dl) but you may get symptoms at higher levels than this. Low blood sugar means there is too much insulin around in your body for the amount of sugar in your blood.

If you don't treat a hypo by eating something containing sugar, your blood sugar may become so low that you become unconscious. This will not cause you permanent damage, nor is it fatal (unless you happen to be in a dangerous situation such as in water or on scaffolding). Even if nobody treated an unconscious hypo, you would come round again. Your body has stores of sugar in your liver and these would be released into your bloodstream to raise your blood sugar — but this would take some time.

Serious note: if you drink alcohol, you *must* eat well. Alcohol lowers your blood sugar partially by blocking this release of sugar from your liver. This means your body will have difficulty in raising your blood sugar to bring you round if you pass out — be careful. Alcohol is covered in detail in Chapter 10.

Very occasionally, hypos that lead to unconsciousness may be accompanied by fits (convulsions). This may be worrying to people watching but there is no evidence that it will do you any permanent brain damage. It is possible that you might hurt yourself if you fall into something such as a piece of furniture, or if you are driving (see Chapter 17 for more detail on driving).

Many people with diabetes find hypos frightening. Some

therefore try to avoid ever getting near a hypo by keeping their blood sugar high. This is not a good idea. Constantly high blood sugars won't make you feel well in the short term — your energy will be low and you will heal slowly, for instance, and this may lead to problems in 20 or 30 years' time.

If you are afraid of hypos, see if you can work out why you are. Have you absorbed fear from other people? Most likely this will be from those who don't have diabetes themselves, since hypos are more worrying to watch (like many things) than to experience. Your parents may be nervous about hypos and so may your clinic staff. If it is someone else's fear, try to leave it with them — you don't have to make it your problem as well.

Maybe you are worried about 'losing control' and behaving in an embarrassing way. Brothers and sisters may take delight in winding you up by telling you bizarre stories about how you behaved. This may be a way of them dealing with the fear, or because they want something from you. Try talking about it — this is easier if you are not embarrassed yourself, and why should you be?

Some people 'use' hypos to get attention and sympathy. People soon get fed up and angry with you if you do this, so you will lose out in the end — not a helpful way to live.

Advice to others

You could suggest to people that they don't ask you questions when you are hypo, but just hand you something sugary (preferably unwrapped). It can be very difficult to get the answer to a question out — your brain may know it, but your mouth won't co-operate. Also, if someone says 'Are you OK?' you are likely to say 'Yes' whether you are or not! All this can be very frustrating so that you may want to shake someone or bash something. This is not the same as being violently aggressive and wanting to hurt someone, and it might be a good idea to explain this to people.

Still, hypos do interfere with what you are doing, so you need to be able to:
● recognize when you are going low
● take steps to put this right
● prevent it from happening too often.

Recognizing hypos

Hypo symptoms vary from person to person and they may alter as you get older or change your type of insulin. These symptoms may include shakiness, sweating, hunger, tiredness, pins and needles around your mouth and lips, blurred vision, lack of concentration, slurring your words, headaches, bad temper, tearfulness, an increased heart rate, and 'leaden' legs. You must learn to recognize your own symptoms.

People around you may notice you going pale or getting a glazed look in your eyes. Ask them what they notice as it will help you to connect this with how you feel at the same time. If your blood sugar level drops very fast, you may, unfortunately, get less warning.

If you go hypo in the night, the early symptoms will usually wake you up, so it is wise to keep something sugary beside your bed. If you wake up with a headache, it may mean that you have been low in the night. It isn't dangerous if you don't wake because your body will release its glucose stores from your liver to raise your blood sugar level in time. By the way, it would take a massive overdose of insulin to kill you — more than a bottle full — so insulin isn't the perfect murder or suicide weapon.

Treating hypos

Fast treatment should restore your blood sugar level to the non-hypo range within minutes. So, as soon as your warning symptoms occur:

● STOP what you are doing!

It is no good thinking 'I'll just finish this first then I'll get something to eat.' Because of your lack of concentration (maybe 'brain-fade' is a good way of putting it), whatever you are doing will take you ages, by which time someone else may have to feed you. Interruptions to deal with hypos can be maddening, but hypos don't just go away if you leave them.

The faster you eat, the faster you can get back to what you want to be doing.

● EAT some sugary carbohydrate!

Pick something that you like and that is easy to carry and to eat. Packets will be difficult to open if you are uncoordinated and shaky; chocolate, if it has been hot, will be messy. You will need 10–20g of carbohydrate to start with. For 10g you need 3 glucose tablets, 2 level teaspoons of honey, jam or sugar, 50ml of Lucozade (there are 50g in a small bottle — work out how many gulps 50ml is), one-third of a can of any fizzy drink (*not* the diet kind!). A fun-sized chocolate bar is more than 10g but less than 20g, usually. Look up the carbohydrate values in the BDA's book *Countdown* to work out how many of different types of sweets equal 10g, if you want.

Glucose tablets are recommended by your clinic because they are easy to carry around and not so nice that you are likely to eat the whole packet, which will probably be more than you need. However, you must choose something you like so that you are inclined to eat it, and will accept it from other people without getting stroppy.

If you don't feel better within five to ten minutes, have another 10–20g of carbohydrate. It is very easy to overtreat yourself since you feel very hungry usually and you may panic about dropping lower still. No great harm will be done if you do eat more than you need, but try not to. Panic can be helped by sitting down and waiting for 5–10 minutes after eating your first 20g. Asking other people to watch the clock helps to calm them too.

You should *always* carry some sort of sugar with you. This way you won't have to rely on someone else having something on them or finding a shop at a time when speed is important (and you may not be clear-headed enough to organize buying something). Carrying sugar on you will also make it easier for others if you are ever found in need of help when hypo.

If you are unsure whether you are hypo or not, you can always check with a blood test. If you find you are having difficulty doing the test, have something to eat before proceeding! You should note that a rush of adrenalin (excitement or fear) may also give you an increased heart rate, the shakes, and sweats. However, adrenalin raises your blood sugar; pre-exam or competition nerves don't mean you are necessarily hypo.

You should also carry some identification on you to tell people that you have diabetes treated with insulin. There are various necklets or bracelets on the market that can be engraved. Medic-Alert ones are also engraved with a telephone number that can be called free worldwide. The enquirer can then obtain relevant details about you and your diabetes. Other systems contain written information slotted into the jewellery. The cheapest way is to get a pet's disc engraved. Hopefully, you can find a design that you don't feel stupid wearing. You may need to explain to your school why you must wear this if they object to jewellery. You should take it off when playing some sports.

Preferably you should also carry a card with your insulin dose and type on it. These have space too for an emergency contact and give the basic treatment for a hypo. These cards can be obtained from the BDA, from the insulin manufacturers, or from your clinic.

You must tell your friends, teachers and workmates about hypos. Don't expect people to be unhelpful or make fun of you — you wouldn't be if someone told you about their asthma, for instance, would you? Other people just need to know what you would like them to do if you are not taking the right steps to rectify a hypo yourself.

You might like to tell them that it will be easier for you to drink something sweet through a straw at this time, as well as what they should feed you and where it is. They also need to know how long recovery takes and that hypos are not dangerous.

You should tell them that if you are unconscious they can put a sugar lump or sweet in your cheek and massage your cheek to dissolve and absorb the sugar. They should not give you liquid if you are 'out' or you might choke. You should mention that you are not short of oxygen, so it does *not* apply that if you don't come round in 4 minutes you will be brain damaged. If in doubt, they should call a doctor or ambulance and say that you have insulin dependent diabetes.

An ambulance person may give you glucose into a vein to bring your blood sugar level up and bring you round; so may a doctor. It is also possible to inject a substance called glucagon. This is a natural substance, not a manufactured drug, which speeds up the proces of your body releasing the glucose you have stored in your liver into your bloodstream.

Glucagon comes in a kit complete with a syringe and needle for an injection under the skin or into a muscle (there is no need to find a vein). It is available on prescription. Your parents might like to have a kit at home, and it would be good to have some around if you are living with friends. Try to get hold of an out-of-date kit so that people can practise putting the stuff together when there is no need to be stressed about it.

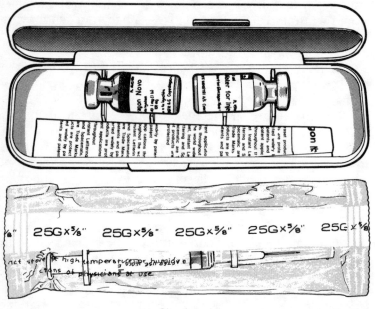

Glucagon kit

After you have been given glucagon, you must have something to eat as soon as you come round. Otherwise, your blood sugar will start to drop again and this time the glucose stores in your liver will be low. If you have been unconscious, you may feel very cold when you come round — your companions should know that you might like a sweater or a blanket. You may also need to pee, have a headache and feel a bit sick, but not everybody feels these things.

You may never need to use glucagon, but it is a very good safety net. Do check that your kit is still in date from time to time and swap it if it has expired.

Preventing hypos

Hypos are more likely to occur if:

- you miss a meal or snack
- you delay a meal — especially lunch if you're on two injections
- you skimp on a meal
- you take heavy exercise without compensating in some way.

How much flexibility you have with the first three of these will vary with your insulin regime, and with what your blood sugar is on any particular day.

Exercise
When you exercise, your muscles use up sugar more rapidly than when they are at rest. Therefore, to prevent hypos you can:

- take extra carbohydrate
- reduce your insulin dose.

To follow the first course, you need to learn how much extra carbohydrate you need for a particular activity. A general guide might be 10–20g of rapidly absorbed carbohydrate before the activity e.g. a fun-sized chocolate bar. If the activity is likely to continue for a long time, take a further 10–20g of slowly absorbed starch at the same time e.g. a wholemeal sandwich; follow this with another 10–20g as well after a couple of hours if still exercising.

Be aware that the effects of exercise may be prolonged, which means you may be hypo many hours after the exercise. Test your blood sugar before you go to bed just in case. If it seems lowish, take another 10–20g of long-acting carbohydrate to see you through the night.

Reducing your insulin dose is the best course of action when you know exercise is planned (providing it doesn't also depend on the weather being suitable!). You will need to work out which insulin to reduce if you are on a combination of short- and long-acting insulins. Usually this will be the short-acting, but it may be both if the exercise is long-lasting. You will also need to work out by how much to reduce your dose. Again, no rules. Some people find that altering it by not more than 2 units at a time gives them a yardstick; others start on a 10 per cent reduction.

If your exercise is strenuous and prolonged, the reductions in your insulin may be considerable (Chapter 11), and you will probably need to increase your carbohydrate intake as well. By the way, exercise hypoglycaemia is not confined to those with diabetes. Long-distance cyclists and marathon runners recognize reaching a 'wall' which can be got through by eating something sweet, or resting until their body catches up with them. You might like to ask a cyclist or runner about this — it may make diabetes feel less 'odd'.

While we're on this subject, very many people without diabetes experience mild hypos; although they may not know what they are, they will know that eating something sweet is what they need to feel better. Ask people about feeling bad-tempered and/or shaky when lunch is delayed!

There isn't always a reason that you can find for hypos, so try not to feel you should know why a hypo happened and don't blame yourself for them. (Though do be honest, at least with yourself, if you could have avoided a hypo.) If you develop a regular pattern of hypos, you may need to talk to the people at the clinic about reducing your insulin or increasing your food intake on a more permanent basis. Growing affects balance too, which comes in later (Chapter 14).

You may not like hypos but they can have positive sides too, sometimes. Some people see dramatic and exciting pictures, colours or shapes when they are hypo, or they may get important personal revelations (and before you ask, the psychedelic drugs do lower your blood sugar too).

You can also use hypos as an excuse to get out of something you don't want to do: not a course of action to be rec-ommended, since manipulating others isn't a good basis for any relationship. It also rubs off on others with diabetes — other people may go away with the impression that all people with diabetes can't go to parties, swim, or whatever else it is you don't happen to enjoy.

Hypos to the extent of being unconscious may take you to hospital. If this happens to you a lot, is there an emotional reason behind it? Do you want to 'escape' for a while and be looked after? Talking about all this with someone can help you to build up more open friendships, which in turn will help to make life more fun outside hospital.

You could try writing a list of the advantages and disadvantages of hypos (be honest!) and see what this looks like. You might like to share this with your family and friends too.

Hypers

'Hypers' mean high blood sugars. It is unfortunate that hypoglycaemia and hyperglycaemia are such similar words since it can get confusing. Blame the Ancient Greeks for this! Technically, hyperglycaemia occurs when your blood sugar is above 11mmol/l (200mg/dl).

You will be hyper when you have not enough insulin in your body, which may happen if:

- your dose of insulin is reduced
- your insulin is not given at all
- you are physically ill
- you are stressed or worried
- you have eaten too much.

It seems to be quite difficult for people without diabetes to understand that it is possible for you to give yourself an incorrect dose of insulin or even genuinely to forget to inject yourself. But we all do both of these things at times, without meaning to be 'difficult' or it having deep emotional significance. You can just forget! So don't feel guilty or stupid if you do either of these things. Don't panic, just work out a way to sort things out later when you realize what you have done.

Illness
If you are ill and do not feel like eating, you may think you should reduce or even stop taking your insulin. Either of these is a recipe for disaster. NEVER stop taking your insulin: ketoacidosis leading to a diabetic coma might happen if you do. Fortunately, this is a much slower process than developing a hypo — you will get the symptoms of high blood sugar (thirst, more trips to the loo, low energy) for several hours before you get anywhere near a coma. However, you must do

something to prevent your balance going haywire. Remember too that if you are ill, your blood sugar is likely to rise anyway, so you may need less food to balance your insulin dose.

Try to read this bit *before* you are actually ill!

If you lose your appetite, feel sick or are vomiting:

1. Take fluids

Try to take your usual grams in liquid form, though don't worry if you can't manage it all since you may need less. Fluids are absorbed in the stomach in considerable amounts even if they are only kept down for a short while. You could use Lucozade, Ribena, fruit juice, soup or milk. Little and often is a good idea — a small glass (don't overface yourself), at hourly intervals maybe. Drink water as well if you are vomiting to replace the fluid you are losing.

2. Test your blood sugar

You may need to do this as often as every two hours. Ask someone to help if you don't feel up to it.

3. Adjust your insulin dose

If your blood sugar is less than 10 mmol/l, continue with your usual dose.

If your blood sugar is between 10 and 12 mmol/l, keep an eye on it and test in another hour's time.

If your blood sugar is greater than 12 mmol/l, increase your quick-acting insulin, probably by 4 units at a time to start with. If your blood sugar is still above 12 mmol/l four hours later, you may need still more clear insulin, and this may mean putting in an extra injection if you are on only two a day. It is wise to discuss illness with your clinic team before it happens since they can give you appropriate guidelines for your insulins.

If you can't sort all this out after a few hours, call the doctor. You don't get any Brownie points for struggling on alone.

Stress

The effects of stress are difficult to measure. It is a bit like 'How long is a piece of string?' If you know you are stressed or worried, meditation or yoga techniques may help. So may tackling and/or changing whatever it is that is bothering you — worrying *won't* help, though. Does it ever?

As with hypos, people without diabetes may also get raised blood sugar levels, for example, before exams, after accidents, or during illness. Obviously they won't go as far up as yours could because their bodies can still produce insulin when required, but it still happens. Many people will admit to feeling sluggish after a very heavy meal, or to feeling a dry mouth before a test.

It may have occurred to you that as exercise lowers your blood sugar, if you are a bit hyper (and not ill) you could go for a run or dig the garden to lower your blood sugar. This is certainly logical thinking but it doesn't always work since it depends *how* high your blood sugar is. If you are producing ketones and using your fat stores for energy, exercise will make this worse. If you are producing ketones (you find this out with a dip stick urine test — sticks will be supplied at your clinic or by your family doctor), taking a little more clear, quick-acting insulin and resting is a better solution.

It is difficult to think of advantages of hypers — except that you will avoid being hy*po*. If you keep your blood sugar always above 10mmol/l, your body may become accustomed to this. You may then feel hypo at, say, 8mmol/l. This isn't a good idea for reasons mentioned already — you won't feel or be fit and you may be storing up problems for yourself in the future.

A few more words about illnesses. You are no more likely than anyone without diabetes to get any other illnesses, unless you are frequently hyper. If your blood sugar is often high, your body won't be able to fight infections so well and healing will take longer. You are also more likely to get unsightly things like boils and it probably won't help acne (which will be helped by a low-fat diet, by the way).

Don't worry about the amount of sugar in medicines. There is probably only 5g in a teaspoonful and it is better to take something and get well more quickly anyway. If you have to go into hospital for anything other than diabetes, hopefully your diabetes care team will also be involved and the ward staff will known something about diabetes. You may need to be assertive if you find you know more about what is right for you than members of staff. Assuming you are not admitted as an emergency, talking to people beforehand may help.

It isn't easy, this constant balancing act. In fact, it is, perhaps, the real burden of having diabetes — you do get used

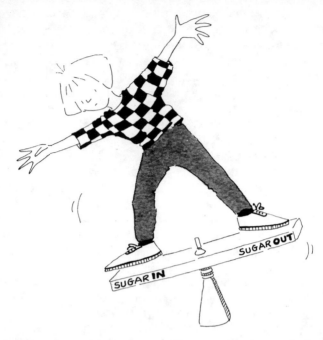

to the blood tests and injections but we all miss not being able to be completely spontaneous sometimes. You may get to feel you can't be bothered and that nothing seems to work anyway. When you do feel like this, arrange to let yourself off the hook for a day and be nice to yourself. This doesn't mean giving up insulin for a day is OK: it isn't. You can't have a total holiday from diabetes ever, but relaxing about it for a while and doing something you really enjoy will help from time to time. Do you have someone around who could do your 'diabetic thinking' for you for a day, once in a while? This might be worth trying.

Chapter 10

More Information on Food

For some people with diabetes, the dietitian is public enemy number one. Dietitians do vary in how easy they are to talk to and how much they know about living with diabetes, but that is true of other people too. They do have a lot of useful information about food and eating, however, so it is worth trying to get to know them so you can use their knowledge to help you with your diabetes.

By the way, you may hear of some foods that will lower blood sugars, particularly guar (a type of gum) and karela, an Indian vegetable. These can be sometimes used by older people with Type II diabetes and do have some effect when diabetes is controlled by diet alone. However, they both taste horrid and won't make much difference to your type of diabetes and your blood sugar levels. No magic for us there!

Eating out

To start with, you really can eat out anywhere you care to. As usual, you will need to pre-plan a bit and educate yourself about which particular carbohydrate is in different or 'foreign' foods you might want to try. Your dietitian and various BDA publications can help here and more places are beginning to put food values on their menus and labels. There is also a move in society generally to go for more healthy low-fat, high-fibre and less-added-sugar types of food. With experience, trial and error, you will learn to guess accurately enough how many grams there are in things.

Indian food is often high in fibre, the flour used may be

made from pulses, and these are also often used as vegetables. Unfortunately, it is also high in fat quite often and Indian desserts are very sweet.

Pizzas contain a lot of carbohydrate but now more places are offering them on a wholemeal base, and there is more 'brown' pasta about.

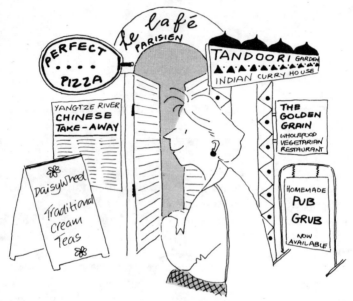

YOU REALLY **CAN** EAT OUT **ANYWHERE** YOU CARE TO....

Greek food is again quite high in fat but may not have much carbohydrate apart from the pitta bread (a white one of these contains 40g of carbohydrate).

Chinese food, apart from the sweet and sour, is low in carbohydrate. You often feel full after all those different dishes but watch out later, you may be low.

Any restaurant dessert may be full of sugar, so think about it. This doesn't mean you should always ask for fresh fruit or cheese and biscuits — it just means 'think about it'. Nor does any of the above mean you should avoid eating different foods; do experiment as much as you like, but thoughtfully.

Many people will try to steer you away from 'junk' food, most of them adults. This is something to learn about, too — some of it is more junky than others. It has its place as it is often fast to buy and to eat and this can be convenient. However, a diet of only junk food will give anyone a lousy complexion and may make anyone, with or without diabetes, fat. Did you know that a milkshake may contain 60g of carbohydrate and 350 calories?

Eating out in someone else's house and in restaurants may mean you have to think about timing, both of injections and of food. There are various solutions you can try, depending on the number and type of injections you have. For instance, you could, if your evening meal is to be later, swap your bedtime snack for dinner/tea-time, perhaps tiding yourself over with a few units of fast-acting insulin; then you could have your full dose and main meal grams later. Altering your meal time an hour or so either way is unlikely to matter very much anyway, unless you are on only one injection a day.

Other people's knowledge of diabetes and food may be limited. It may even be wrong if they are expecting you to be like granny who has Type II diabetes, is on 'diet alone' treatment and is overweight. If the worst comes to the worst and you find after you have injected your usual insulin dose, that you are presented with a carbohydrate-free meal, you may just have to vanish to the loo to eat the emergency supply of sugar you are, of course (!), carrying with you. This sort of thing does tend to spoil a meal out, so a few words when you are invited out is worth the bother. Don't forget, if you feel you need more carbohydrate, you can always ask for bread, or drink something containing sugar.

Then there is the 'Where am I going to inject myself?' dilemma. If you feel happier departing to the bathroom or toilet, by all means do so, but this can have drawbacks. In a restaurant, the loos can be dark, poky, unclean, or, occasionally, non-existent. Also, you may return to your table to find the meal has been delayed for an hour.

Some people think there is a stigma or disgrace attached to injections or they may make some people feel 'green'. It is more important how *you* feel. Diabetes is not something to be ashamed of, or to hide. You will often find people are very interested to learn about diabetes from you (and that is a help to all of us in the future).

If you don't want to explain, few people will notice a discreet under-the-table injection anyway. Some sites are less obvious than others — there is no harm in injecting through your trousers if this is easier. If you want to be open, and you can say it gently, try the line, 'I have to do this but you don't have to watch' or something similar that sounds right for you. Getting over the hump of injecting in public, if it is one, frequently makes people feel better about themselves and their diabetes — so it is worth trying to do this.

Parties and alcohol

At parties there is usually a variety of food around so you can take your pick when you want to eat. If you are disco-ing, that uses up energy so you may need more food, a fruit juice, or a non-diet fizzy drink. There is no reason why you shouldn't stay up all night if you want to, but you may need extra food, being active rather than sleeping, and you will have to think about coping with the following day!

Now, what to drink? Slimline drinks are becoming more widely available, fortunately, but what if there aren't any? If you want a soft drink, you may have to resort to soda or mineral water, perhaps with a dash of squash, or a tomato juice — and a protest to the organizers.

On to *alcohol* . . . no, it isn't banned, but there are things you need to know.

- Alcohol lowers your blood sugar, so you *must* eat when drinking. Don't count the carbohydrate in the alcoholic drink — ignore it. You could alternate booze with a fruit juice to give carbohydrate, or with a slimline drink if you are eating crisps.
- Avoid 'diet' beers. They are very high in alcohol, sugary carbohydrate — and price!
- Sweet wines, ports, sweet sherries and liqueurs also contain a lot of sugary carbohydrate. To lessen their effect on your blood sugar, it is best to use them as a small glass after a high-fibre meal.
- Don't drink on an empty stomach — have a high-fibre snack before you start. (This is a good idea for people without diabetes too; alcohol lowers everyone's blood sugars.)
- Alcohol contains a lot of calories — it makes you fat without providing any nourishment.

- NEVER, EVER drink and drive, not even one drink.
- Symptoms of hypos and drunkenness can be similar. Carry or wear some ID in case the police think you are 'drunk & disorderly'!

Being drunk with a hypo is the one time when the hypo may be dangerous, as the alcohol will prevent your stores of glucose from getting into your bloodstream. Do check your blood sugar before you go to bed after a boozy evening — or eat something anyway, just in case the drink makes doing the test difficult!

Because alcohol slows down all the processes in your body, small doses of it make you feel more relaxed. However, if you drink a lot, your brain has to work harder just to keep you awake. If you then stop drinking, your brain continues to over-react for a while, so you get nervous and shaky until you get another drink — this is the 'DTs' and means you are addicted to alcohol.

The long-term effects of heavy drinking, apart from being addicted, include getting fat; damaging your stomach, kidneys, heart, liver and brain; sexual difficulties; high blood pressure; and depression. Alcohol is also passed into a developing baby and can damage its growth — so don't drink if you are pregnant.

Quite a lot of negatives. Getting drunk doesn't make you tall, rich, strong, handsome, smart, witty, sophisticated or sexy. So do think about how much you drink.

Eating too much or too little

Getting back to food, people who do not feel good about themselves may develop extreme eating patterns. This may mean being overweight if you eat too much, or developing anorexia nervosa if you eat too little. Both of these can make your life a nightmare, with or without diabetes.

Overeating
Any calories you eat that are not converted to energy and used up are stored under your skin as fat. On average, fat people die sooner than thin people and are more prone to heart disease. It is not a good idea to be fat and have diabetes since there are

then two ways in which you are more likely to get heart disease.

You can diet while you take insulin but you will need to go and talk to a dietitian to find a safe and effective reducing diet that will fit in with your system of insulin injections. Crash diets are unbalanced for anyone. They don't provide you with enough calories to keep you fit, and the main thing you lose is water, so they don't produce a lasting loss of weight. Overall, the best permanent and effective way of losing weight is to develop a new relationship with food.

One way to start is to keep a food diary (honestly — it is no good saying 'that wasn't a typical day'!) and write down for a week all the things you eat, and when, and what else you were doing. Then take a look at this and see when you eat more — do you nibble when worried, for instance, or when you are with certain people? When you see a pattern you can try to change it to a 'thin' pattern.

Things that go with a 'thin' pattern of eating include always sitting down to eat, and eating slowly. Small meals help too: large meals expand your stomach and you may then feel hungry just because you now have a large 'gap' to fill. Trying to lose weight on your own is often more difficult; your dietitian might help you to get a group together.

While we're on being overweight, teenagers go through a growth spurt, particularly boys. At that time you may need more food and more insulin. You need to watch out that this level of food and insulin intake is cut back later if necessary when you have stopped growing; otherwise, you may put on extra weight. Don't forget that exercise is an important part of slimming down, using up those extra calories.

Anorexia nervosa

This is a serious condition which is currently more common in young women than in young men. If you are anorexic, you think you are fat when you are not and become obsessed with slimming, starving yourself to a dramatic loss of weight. There is a related condition known as *bulimia* where, after every (often large) meal, you force yourself to vomit before the food can be absorbed in your stomach.

Both these conditions lead to rapid weight loss along with other damage to your body. This includes periods stopping, hair falling out, and skin drying out and flaking off. The vomiting means that stomach juices are often present in the mouth, which may cause mouth ulcers (sores) and damage the teeth. If not checked, sufferers could eventually starve to death. With diabetes as well, dangers of hypos, ketoacidosis and kidney failure are made larger. This isn't a way of avoiding insulin injections.

The causes for these eating disorders may be emotional. Perhaps girls do not want to grow up and develop a 'womanly' shape. They may be influenced by something or somebody outside themselves, like thinking they are fatter than their friends or that they don't look like magazine models who they think are an ideal shape.

Unfortunately, people with anorexia or bulimia often will not admit anything is wrong and will try to hide the fact that they are not eating or that they are vomiting after eating. As you can probably gather, they are very unhappy and may need psychiatric help to get better. (A psychiatrist is a doctor who specializes in treating mental or emotional problems.)

If you think you may have either of these problems, do try to talk to someone about them. If you don't want people to know, there are various self-help associations you can contact — try your local Citizens Advice Bureau or library for information, or the telephone directory.

When you feel fed up with having diabetes, you may be tempted to have a 'binge' on food — that is, to eat a large amount of food over quite a short time, say six packets of chocolate biscuits or a whole box of chocolates, or several hamburgers. Mind you, people who don't have diabetes binge too, but people seldom remark on this! So if you sometimes binge, don't think you are peculiar, or the only person who ever does this, and there is no need to feel guilty.

If you do binge, try seeing if there is a pattern. When do you do it? How do you feel then? It may be worth looking at what else is happening in your life that you don't like, to see whether you can change anything. Anyway, everyone is entitled to enjoy a binge sometimes, so long as it doesn't become a habit!

Chapter 11

School and Sport

After diagnosis

If you had time off school when diabetes was diagnosed, it may feel strange the first time you go back to school. Even if you haven't had time off, you may be a bit nervous about what to say to people and how they will react. Please don't decide that you don't want anyone to know about your diabetes — that will just make huge barriers between you and others and you will feel very isolated.

Diabetes isn't anything to be ashamed of, nor is it something you should feel you have to hide. It isn't anyone's fault you have diabetes, and diabetes is neither infectious nor messy. Diabetes doesn't leave you incapable of anything either, so don't dramatize it. You will know by now that you do need constant awareness, but you are not physically, intellectually, emotionally, or spiritually inferior (or superior) to people without diabetes.

You will find that most other people at school don't know much about diabetes and they are likely to be very interested in the new knowledge you have. They will also be impressed with how you do blood tests and injections. If you feel you would enjoy it, you could offer to talk to your class (or even the whole school?) about diabetes and you could bring in your diabetic 'equipment' to show everybody. They will probably also be interested to hear your new knowledge about food, too. If you would find giving a talk to a group difficult, your diabetes specialist nurse could perhaps come to school and give a talk.

Your school teachers will need to know what having diabetes means to your school life. They particularly need to know about hypos and how to treat them. Ideally they should keep your favourite hypo remedy in their desks; it isn't very useful if the only sugar is in the school office, which may be miles away. They need to know that you may need to eat in class and during exams and before a games period. They also shouldn't keep you in after school without warning — but this isn't an excuse for you breaking school rules!

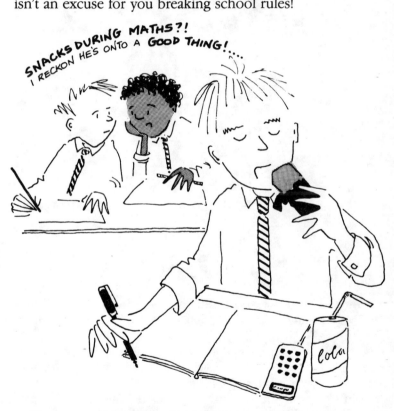

Your parent(s) will probably want to arrange to see your teachers, and your diabetes nurse may also do so. It may be a good idea to talk to the school meals staff if appropriate and people need to know that you will need to eat lunch on time. All the staff and other pupils may need reminding that diabetes is not catching!

Try not to let diabetes influence your choice of lunches at school. Diabetes is not a reason for changing what you did before you were diagnosed. The choice of whether you have school dinners, sandwiches, or go home should be influenced by what you prefer and what is easiest.

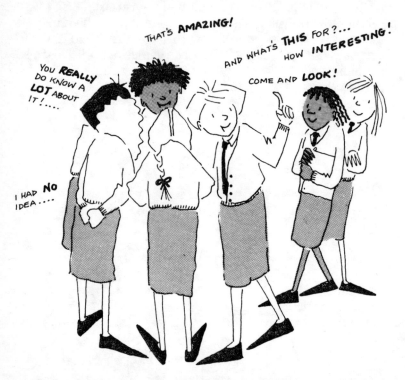

If you do blood tests or injections at school, you may find that using the medical room is preferred by either you or the school staff. Hopefully, you can have an open discussion about this, but you may need to negotiate a compromise if teachers are worried, for instance, about syringes or insulin pens being left in your desk.

You can participate in any activities that are going on and take part in any trips or outings. You will sometimes have to do some pre-planning, as ever, and it is wise for your friends and teachers to know about hypos and how to help you if it becomes necessary. You may find other people watch over you a lot at first, so you may need to mention gently that you don't need this.

For yourself, please don't use diabetes as an excuse to get out of doing things, or to get 'sympathy' — that is manipulation and won't, in the long run, make you or others feel good. Hypos are not a reason to go home from school! Bear in mind that when you are looking for a job or college place, a good school attendance record is a great recommendation.

There is no reason why you can't go away to school if you have diabetes. It would be a good idea in this case to make contact with the diabetic specialist and team closest to your school in case you need them in term time, as well as being on the books of your clinic at home.

Sport

You and others will need to know that you may need to eat something sugary before doing sport, and perhaps during it too. No sports are totally banned to people with diabetes, except that in the UK you can't have a full motor racing licence or get a sub-aqua certificate. It is probably not wise to go swimming alone, but that is true for those without diabetes too. You need to try to avoid hypothermia (getting very cold) as this can be bad news if mixed with a hypo. One tip: if you are out on a long walk, splitting your food supplies between you and your friend is sensible, in case your rucksack drops off a rock!

If you are trying a new sport, ask yourself, 'If I develop a hypo while doing this, how would I organize taking some sugar? If it would be difficult to take sugar, would I be a danger to myself or put anyone else at risk?' With pre-planning, experimenting and talking to others with diabetes, you will be able to do any sport you want. There is a book by John Betteridge, *Sport for Diabetics* (Black, 1988), which you might like to read.

All over the world there are professional sportsmen and women who have insulin dependent diabetes. Their sports range from football to ice-dancing via golf, cricket, speedway racing and hill-climbing (in cars). Gary Mabbutt, who plays football for Spurs and England, has diabetes; so does Randy Mamola, the American motor bike racer.

As a final point for this chapter, you might like to mention to your friends and colleagues that having diabetes doesn't change you into something else; and though it is basically your responsibility how you live with your diabetes, you would appreciate their help if a hypo ever catches you unawares.

Chapter 12

Clinically Speaking

The words 'diabetic clinic' mean different things in different parts of the country. Depending on your age when you were diagnosed and your local facilities, the clinic doctor you see may be a paediatrician (a doctor who specializes in children). This doctor may specialize further in diabetes or treat children with other conditions as well. So when you turn up for an appointment you *may* be just with others with diabetes, or you may not.

The same goes for seeing a physician (a doctor specializing in medical rather than surgical conditions in adults) — s/he may just see people with diabetes, or not. In this case, as there are many adults with diabetes (mostly Type II diabetes), the clinic you attend is likely to be devoted to diabetes on the days you go, but the clients will be of all ages, possibly from 13 upwards.

Some places now have diabetes centres which may be part of the main hospital or in a separate building. The number of these centres is increasing all the time and they are often more 'user friendly' than a huge out-patient clinic where you might be herded about for several hours.

Adolescent clinics are now being set up too in some places, which means you will be with people of a similar age to yourself. Ideally there will be some clinics jointly run by the paediatrician and the physician so you won't suddenly have to transfer to a group of staff you don't know when you get older, which can be a bit unnerving.

It is important to go to a clinic if you want to take care of yourself. As you get older, a yearly check-up may be enough, but if you are still growing, you will probably be given an appointment more frequently. The clinic will probably weigh you and measure your height. They will test your urine for protein — this is an indicator of kidney damage if it is present. They may want you to do a blood test as you would at home to check you are doing this properly.

They may take a sample of blood (probably from a vein) to do an HbAlc test. (Sometimes a 'fructosamine' test is used, which is similar.) The HbAlc test gives an indication of what your balance has been like over the past six weeks or so. Glucose sticks to your red blood cells and the test measures the average of how much has stuck over a period of time. If you have this test done, do ask to know the result and for an explanation of what the number means — and then ask for help in altering (usually reducing) it if necessary.

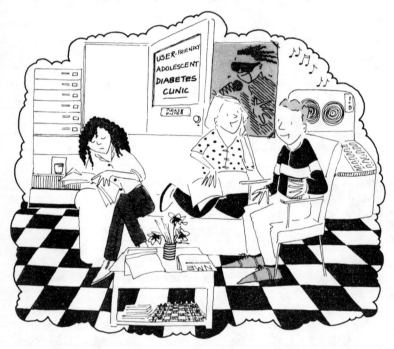

The clinic will also give you regular eye checks — usually annually, but maybe not until a year or two after you have been diagnosed. If you have to have drops in your eyes for this, they do sting a bit and blur your vision for some hours afterwards — don't drive in this state and, if it is very sunny, dark glasses might help. The drops widen your pupils (the hole in the centre of your eyes). Your pupils usually get smaller in bright light, but the drops prevent them from doing this for a while, so your eyes will be very 'sensitive' to light until the drops wear off.

Sometimes the back of your eye may be photographed so that a record can be kept of any changes from one year to the next. The use of these retinal cameras is getting more widespread. As explained in Chapter 7, these eye examinations are to detect any damage to the back of your eye (the retina) which can be treated if picked up early, before it can damage your sight.

Most clinics have a dietitian available whom you can see if you want food information. There might also be a chiropodist around who can look at your feet — prevention is better than cure for any foot problems. As you get older, your blood pressure will probably be checked too. Hopefully, there will be people on the team whom you can talk to about how you feel and about anything in any part of your life that is bothering you.

People sometimes say that they hate going to the clinic and that it is a waste of time. If you start to feel like that, there are things that you can do about it — other than just 'dropping out' and not going at all, which won't help your health in the long term. To start with, think about and write down what you really dislike at the clinic, and what is good there. Also, think about whether you want to go there on your own or with a parent and/or friend. If you do go with someone else, do you want to see the clinic staff together or separately?

Then think about what would make the clinic a more attractive place to visit. Would music help? What about a coffee machine? Magazines? People near your own age? Would an evening clinic be more convenient? What about if the chairs were 'easy' chairs arranged in a circle? These are only a few ideas — you will probably think of others as well. Then, whom do you find easiest in the clinic to talk to? (Come on, they are not *all* ogres!) Try asking them (the diabetes specialist nurse is often a good person to start this conversation with) whether it would be possible to introduce some changes.

Section C

Growing Up

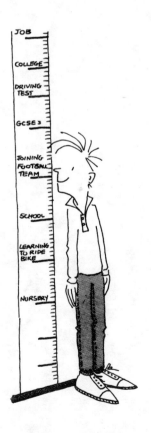

Chapter 13

Parents, Relatives and Friends

Relationships with other people are likely to be the most interesting and the most difficult part of being an adult. They will also be the most difficult part of growing up. Sometimes you may feel pulled in different directions by other people and this may create problems for you and for them. Diabetes, as it is part of your life, will have its effect on you and others too. However, do beware of seeing diabetes as a monster and blaming it for everything that is difficult in your life.

Most people know very little about diabetes. Sometimes what they do know can be incorrect. You will need to decide how much you want to tell people about your diabetes (and about anything else that is part of you), and this probably won't be the same for everyone with diabetes. Anyway, the amount of information you want to share will vary at different times and will depend on whom you are talking to.

Some people you talk to will have only a mild interest in diabetes, both yours and in general. Others will be so curious that it may be difficult to handle, and you will wish they would shut up! Hopefully people will be interested in you as a person, rather than a set of symptoms.

Friends who don't (or won't) understand your diabetes, and try to influence you to do things that may make you ill, don't have your best interests at heart and are immature and selfish — these are 'friends' you can do without.

Having diabetes means that you have to take it into consideration whatever you do — if you try to ignore diabetes, it has unpleasant ways of getting back at you and disrupting your life. However, it is nothing to be ashamed of, feel guilty about, apologize for or hide. If having diabetes makes you feel different at times, you may feel resentful and angry. You may then find that you take this out on other people, by bullying them or being aggressive, and so getting into arguments at home, school or work.

If this sort of thing has ever happened to you, you probably found afterwards that you don't end up feeling very good. People may not understand, when this happens, why you feel this way, so they may react in ways that make you feel even more left out and angry than ever. It is OK to be angry, but try to use that energy positively — don't turn it against yourself or others.

By the way, all teenagers go through mood swings: you may feel on top of the world one minute and in the depths of despair a few moments later. This is part of becoming an adult. It doesn't necessarily mean you are hypo or hyper, though other people may try to label any of your moods as due to diabetes. There is always a blood test if you want to check!

You and your family

Sometimes the people you live with may seem to put up the biggest barriers to you growing up and becoming independent. If you live with your parents, one or both of them may feel it is their fault (and feel guilty) that you have diabetes. If one or both of them has relatives with diabetes, they may believe they have passed diabetes on to you. This *isn't* true: your diabetes isn't anybody's fault. However, these feelings may make parents over-protective. This can be very frustrating when you want to learn to live your own life and make your own decisions.

Parents are people too: they are not from another galaxy. If you are stubborn about the way you handle diabetes, it may be hard for adults to hand over responsibility for your diabetes to you. If you are awkward about your diabetes, they are more likely to treat you like a child, since they won't have confidence that you know what you are doing.

Just as you sometimes feel that you can't do anything right, so do adults and parents. They get into the habit of asking if you've done your injection or have sugar with you every time you go out, and you get into the habit of saying 'yes', whether you have or not! Nagging is annoying but it does mean that people care about you. Do try to talk openly about what is bugging you. Using someone as a 'go-between' (friends, relatives, or even someone at the clinic) may make a conversation easier.

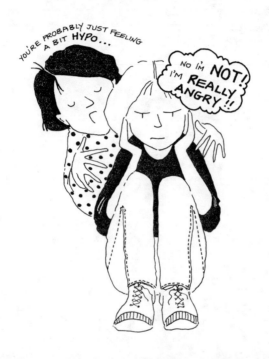

You might like to show this statement to some people: 'I find it very irritating (perhaps insulting) if people assume I am hypo when I am showing a strong emotion (such as anger).'

You may feel at times that being dependent on insulin injections spoils your personal independence. You can see it like that if you want but, unless we go and live on an uninhabited island, we are all dependent on others sometimes. Even on your island you would be dependent on your surroundings so don't see all dependence as a 'bad' thing and restriction.

A few points about growing up:

- your diabetes is yours, not anyone else's
- think about when you would like to go to the clinic alone
- being a teenager doesn't last for ever: most people have survived it (including your parents)
- don't mislay your sense of humour, even if others seem to have lost theirs at times.

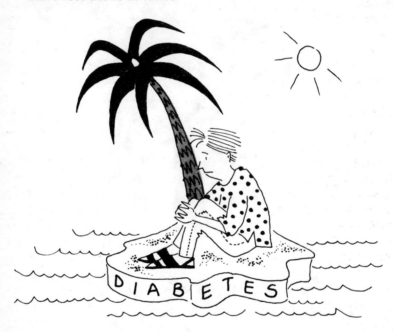

Chapter 14

Puberty

The dictionary defines puberty as the 'beginning of sexual maturity'. If you are wondering when sexual maturity ends, that is probably when you die! The part we are talking about is the beginning, when your glands and hormones start to become active and your body changes into its adult shape.

Sometimes puberty may be delayed in young people who have diabetes, particularly if your blood sugar levels have been high or you were diagnosed just before puberty. However, puberty happens over a wide range of ages in teenagers in general, so try not to worry or feel you are out of step with the rest of your friends and classmates. Your doctor can reassure you if you feel that would help.

For some people it is very difficult to avoid wide swings in blood sugar levels when all this other glandular and hormone activity is going on as well. These growth and sexual hormones may act counter to insulin; that is, they may *raise* your blood sugar. Try not to worry about this: the time when balance is difficult, even if this lasts for a year or two, is unlikely to harm you in the long term. Accepting that things may be uneven for a while will mean that you won't add stress as another factor which might raise your blood sugar.

If you are female, you may find your balance changes a day or two before your period starts. If you ask women without diabetes, you quite often find that they will get 'the munchies' before period comes on. If this happens to you, you may find it is because your blood sugar is low (this may be true for women without diabetes, too) — then you will need to decide whether you have a little less insulin or a bit more food at this time of the month.

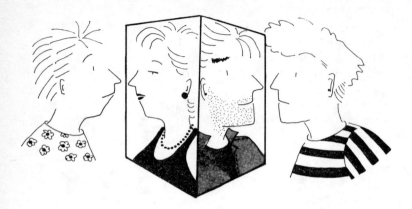

On the other hand, if you suffer from pre-menstrual tension (PMT), you may feel stressed and not have much energy to move about, so your blood sugars may be higher. Once again, you will need to find your own pattern and how you want to remedy any changes in blood sugar levels. Until you settle into a fairly regular monthly cycle, you may have to deal with a different pattern each month, unfortunately.

If you are concerned that your body is the 'wrong' shape or size in any way (and most young people think this at some time) take a trip to your local swimming pool and study the range of bodies there. They are very varied.

Sex

There is a lot of rubbish talked and written about sex. People may mix up their views on sex with their religious or moral views (the way they think you 'ought' to behave). This can lead to very fixed ideas about what is 'right' and 'wrong' in general, instead of allowing people to find what is right and wrong for *them*.

Certainly you should never forget that sex is a life force and involves very powerful feelings. That said, there are no universal standards of what is 'right' and 'wrong'. In discovering what is right for you, there is one useful yardstick — if you or your partner are not finding the activity pleasurable, forget it! And don't confuse sex and love. Ideally you get these two together with the same person, but don't rush into long-term commitments until you are sure.

It may have occurred to you that sex is a form of exercise, so those of us with diabetes need to think about food too. Make sure food is readily to hand. By the way, if Lucozade is your chosen hypo remedy, it can be difficult to get the top off the bottle when you are hypo and sexually excited, so put an elastic band round the lid to help your grip. Perhaps buying your partner a box of chocolates could be useful at times too!

Yes, you do need to tell anyone with whom you have a close friendship, sexual or not, about diabetes. Eating together may be a way to start the conversation naturally. Diabetes isn't something to be ashamed of and you shouldn't assume that it will turn people off. Any relationship needs to be based on mutual acceptance of whole people — accepting your diabetes is obviously part of this. If someone can't or won't accept the whole of you, it is better to know sooner rather than later. This doesn't mean it won't be painful and hurt, but think enough of yourself to see it as their loss as well as yours.

Diabetes is no bar to long-term relationships or marriage. You will have the same pitfalls and traumas in this as the rest of the world. Just one point, diabetes doesn't cause relationships to break up, but it may act as a focus for incompatibility (not getting on with someone). For instance, if your partner thinks you should not inject yourself 'in

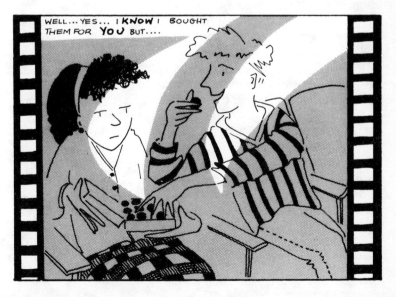

public', beware — does s/he really accept diabetes as an OK part of you?

Diabetes shouldn't affect your sexual performance in any way. However, if your blood sugar is high you may need frequent trips to the loo, and if you are hypo, for men, things that go up will come down!

Contraception

Both men and women with diabetes are fertile, so diabetes is not a reliable method of contraception — don't use it!

Unplanned and unwanted pregnancies are bad news for everyone involved, perhaps more so if you have diabetes and are female (see the later section on pregnancy). All currently available methods of contraception are suitable for use by people with diabetes. You need to consider your personal preferences and any other medical history you have.

Many women with diabetes take the Pill with no problems. The hormones in the Pill may cause your insulin requirements to change a little (either up or down) so it would be wise to monitor this. The hormones contained in the Pill are those produced during pregnancy, so your body believes you are pregnant and won't produce an egg to be fertilized, so you won't get pregnant.

It now seems that, if you take a high-dose pill continually for several years, you have an increased risk of cervical cancer (cancer of the neck of your womb) — this applies to all women. So it is recommended that you take the 'mini', progesterone-only Pill. The only drawback with this Pill is that you must take it at the same time every day of the course to be totally protected from an unwanted pregnancy. As a system, women with diabetes could always take it with their evening insulin injection. The Pill is available only on prescription, from your family doctor or a family planning clinic.

Barrier methods of contraception may not seem as convenient as the Pill but they can be equally reliable and may protect you from sexually transmitted diseases as well as pregnancy. If you don't have sex regularly, barrier methods may be a better choice than taking the Pill all the time.

For women, if you choose a cap or diaphragm, it must be

fitted properly. Caps are made of rubber with the rim made springy by the insertion of metal wire. They fit over the neck of the womb to prevent the sperm meeting the egg. Caps must be used with spermicide, a chemical cream which inactivates or kills sperm. It is *not* enough to use a spermicide on its own, just in case you have seen them on sale in chemists and thought this would avoid organizing a doctor's appointment.

The most readily available barrier method, the only safe method you can get without seeing a doctor/clinic, and the only (at the moment) contraceptive used by men, is the condom or sheath. (They also have dozens of 'slang' names by which they are known, e.g. Johnnies and French Letters, to mention just two.) With the advance of AIDS as a fatal, sexually transmitted disease, condoms are on sale not only in chemists, but also in supermarkets, garages and from slot machines.

If you participate in a male homosexual relationship, you should also use condoms, since AIDS is more common amongst male homosexuals. It is also more common amongst people who inject 'illegal' drugs. If you are in a heterosexual relationship and you are unsure of your partner's previous sex life, make sure you use a condom, even if you are using another form of contraceptive — that will only prevent you getting pregnant; it won't prevent you getting AIDS. If anyone won't use a condom, do you really want to have sex with this person?

On the subject of AIDS, do get reliable facts about how it is spread, and don't believe any press or public hysteria. Certainly, the fewer sexual partners you have, the lower your risk. You can't catch AIDS from working alongside anyone who is HIV positive (that means they are carrying cells in their blood which may develop into AIDS at a later date) or has AIDS, or from public toilet seats — to quote just two of the many myths around.

If you are worried that you may have been in contact with AIDS through a sexual partner, or in contact with any other sexually transmitted disease, you can get checked over at the special clinic at your local hospital — you don't have to tell anyone else that you are going there, or be referred by another doctor. There are treatments for syphilis, gonorrhoea and non-specific urinary infections and the sooner you get treatment, the less damage these diseases will do to you.

If you get any unusual discharge (a leak of liquid) from your penis or vagina, particularly if it is smelly or itchy, do go and seek medical advice. There is no need to be embarrassed; the doctor will not judge your behaviour — s/he is there to help cure whatever it is. If your blood sugar levels are out of balance, you are more likely to get urinary infections.

To get contraceptive advice and help, you can go to your diabetic team or your GP, but you don't have to ask either of them if you don't want to. The phone number and address of your nearest Family Planning Clinic will be in your local phone book. To be seen without reference to your parents or guardians, you have to be aged 16 or older at present. Their advice and treatment is free. If you feel people don't understand about diabetes (for instance, they may say you shouldn't take the Pill), shop around for another clinic or doctor who does understand.

Both men and women with diabetes can be sterilized, but you must realize that this is *not* reversible. This may be a contraception method to consider when you are sure you have had as many children as you want (which may be none, of course). It is not something to undertake without very serious thought and discussion on an emotional level. Even though the operations are now very quick and fairly easy, that is just the physical side.

You can get more information from the Family Planning Association and from books, perhaps in a library. To finish with, here are a few things to remember:

- You CAN get pregnant if you do it standing up.
- You CAN get pregnant if you are on your period.
- You CAN get pregnant the first time.
- You CAN get pregnant even if you wash straight away.
- You CAN get pregnant even if your partner's penis doesn't enter your vagina.
- You CAN get pregnant if your partner is being careful and withdrawing before he comes.
- You CAN get pregnant if you don't come.

Chapter 15

Do You Want to Have Children?

Obviously the timing of this decision will be affected by many things but, for a beginning, you might like to know the risks of your children also getting diabetes. If the father has insulin dependent diabetes (I.D.D.) 1 in 20 of his children will have it too. If the mother has I.D.D. 1 in 100 of her children will have it too. (Nobody knows at the moment why there is this difference between men and women.) If both parents have I.D.D. the chances of the children having it are higher. If one parent and one brother or sister have I.D.D. 1 in 10 of any other children will also have it.

All these figures don't tell you what will happen to *you* though. You will have to weigh this up for yourself because no one can tell you definitely whether *your* child or children will develop diabetes. You also need to consider that if your child did develop diabetes, would this be a reason to decide not to have children at all?

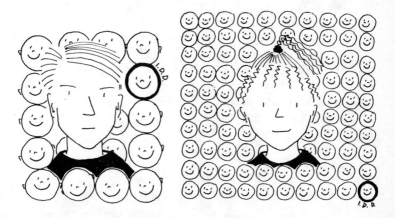

Before insulin was discovered, nobody developing diabetes as a child would have lived long enough to have children. Even after insulin treatment, say before the Second World War, many women died when they were pregnant, or the child died just before birth. For some reason, babies of mothers with diabetes grew very large just before they were due to be born and sometimes they died before or soon after birth. This seems to be related to high blood sugar levels during pregnancy, which means that nowadays, with blood glucose monitoring being easy to carry out at home, horror stories of women with diabetes having huge babies or not being able to have babies at all should be a thing of the past.

From the 1950s, survival of mother and child started to improve, though it was noticed that more of the babies born to mothers with diabetes seemed to have the kinds of damage that were formed when the foetus (the baby growing in the womb) was only 4–6 weeks into its life in the womb. These problems are called 'congenital malformations' and include things like spina bifida.

Things are very different now, so don't let that put you off having children if you want to. It is now realized that, for a woman with diabetes planning a pregnancy, it is important to get your blood sugars as close to the normal range as you can *before* you try to conceive. This way you will maximize your chances of having a healthy baby. You would be wise to go to a hospital that has expert doctors who are interested in pregnancy and diabetes. Some diabetes centres now have pre-pregnancy counselling, so this is worth checking out. It is not known at present, if the parent with diabetes is the man, whether his blood sugar levels also affect the chances of having a healthy baby.

If you keep your blood sugar levels under strict control during your pregnancy, and providing there are no other non-diabetic related problems, there is now no reason why you shouldn't carry your baby to 'full-term' — usually 40 weeks in the womb. (Previously, babies were often delivered early, perhaps by a Caesarean, just in case they got too large.) You will need to attend a hospital frequently, perhaps once a month to begin with, then once a fortnight after six months of pregnancy; but now there should be no need to be admitted to hospital, unless there are non-diabetic problems, until the end of your pregnancy.

You are likely to need much more insulin during pregnancy — doses often double by the end — though some women need less insulin in the first three months. Labour (the time your baby is actually being born) takes up a lot of energy so your blood sugar and insulin levels will need to be watched closely. Because of this, you would not be advised to try to have your baby at home: much better to have hospital back-up and experts in birth and diabetes close at hand.

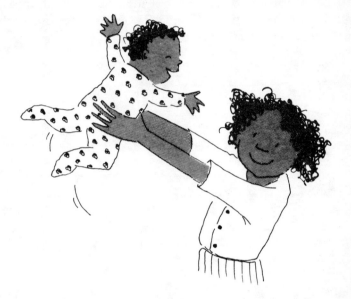

There is plenty of information about diabetes and pregnancy around, so do find out as much as you can before you decide to have a baby. Talking to other women with diabetes who have had children is a good way to start — your diabetic team or the BDA can help with contacts when you need them.

After the birth, your insulin dose will quickly (within a day or two) return to its pre-pregnancy levels. Your baby may be born with a low blood sugar and will be watched closely for the first 12 hours or so, so that any problems arising can be quickly treated. Women with diabetes can certainly breast-feed if they want to. Just one thing to remember, though: if you feed your baby when your blood sugar is low, it won't get as much nourishment and may want feeding again quite soon. Feed yourself first, and then feed the baby (you may need to ignore cries for a few minutes!). While you are breast-feeding you may need more food and less insulin — work it out by trial and error again, with advice from your diabetic team.

Overall, don't go into a pregnancy without a considerable amount of thought. It will require a lot of self-discipline for at least a year to keep a tight balance on your blood-sugar levels. That done, you can be confident that you can produce a healthy baby.

One final word; at the other extreme, women with diabetes can have abortions. But for anyone this can be very distressing and is better avoided. See Chapter 14 on contraception — that is a much better way.

Chapter 16

Different Types of Drugs

Illegal drugs

You may, as you get older and your social life gets wider, find yourself somewhere where drugs are being circulated. A cigarette passed round from person to person is likely to contain cannabis (also known as pot, grass, hash, or marijuana) and may also contain heroin (junk, smack, H, or horse). Please do refuse this or any other unknown powders or pills you may be offered.

Remember that:

- all these drugs are addictive — you may get to depend on them
- a little *will* do you harm
- smoking or sniffing drugs is just as dangerous as injecting them
- drug users who inject into a vein are at great risk from infections — particularly AIDS and hepatitis, which will kill you
- drugs cost a lot — both money and your health.

Glue or solvent sniffing (that is, breathing in the chemicals in glue, petrol or aerosol sprays) makes you feel light-headed ('high'), sometimes a bit like alcohol. This is a very dangerous pastime since the chemicals severely damage your brain, liver, lungs, kidneys and bones, and this leads to your death. Sniffing from plastic bags can cause death by suffocation.

Diabetically, drugs will have an effect on your blood sugar. 'Uppers' (pep pills) may raise or lower it. Cannabis may lower your blood sugar and also give you a craving for sweet things. Heroin and cocaine slow down the passage of food through your guts which may cause your blood sugars to rise as you absorb more of what you eat. Since all these drugs will have an effect on your state of mind, you may not know if you are hypo or hyper. They also confuse your memory — you may not know if you have given yourself insulin or food, or how much of either.

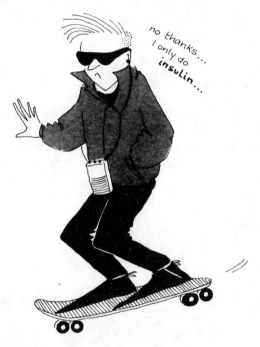

Illegal drugs are not glamorous or macho. They are sordid, expensive and, in the end, they kill you. You already know that being dependent on insulin injections is a burden at times — think about what it would be like to be dependent on some other substance as well. If you are already involved with the drug scene, seek professional help as soon as you can.

You should be aware that some young people with diabetes have been stopped by the police and questioned about the insulin syringes they were carrying. This is another reason for carrying and/or wearing some sort of ID stating that you have diabetes. Should you be taken to a police station, get the police to contact a member of your diabetic team to vouch for you.

Do remember to dispose of your used syringes and blood testing lancets carefully. This is to avoid causing the dustbin man pain if he sticks one in his finger when he empties your bin and to prevent them from being used by drug addicts. There are clippers available free that will cut off and safely store a used needle. Or you can put used syringes and lancets in a soft drink can, seal it when full and then put it in a dustbin. Some hospitals may give you a plastic bin with a lid that you can return to the hospital when it is full and they will burn it for you.

Smoking

Hopefully most people now know that smoking (cigarettes, cigars or pipes filled with tobacco) is not a 'good thing' to do to yourself, or to other people. To give some more details:

The tar in tobacco smoke irritates your air passages which makes them narrower and increases mucus production in an attempt to help the irritation. Your lungs become unable to get rid of the mucus or the dirt and bacteria that also get in them. This leads to 'smoker's cough', which is really a kind of bronchitis (an infection of the tubes leading to your lungs), which means your lungs are also more prone to infections.

The chemical nicotine in tobacco is addictive (once you've started, you keep wanting more of it) and acts on your brain and nervous system. Nicotine makes your heart beat faster and narrows your blood vessels, contributing to heart and circulatory disease. Diabetes also contributes to heart and circulatory diseases, so you are loading the dice against yourself if you smoke as well as having diabetes. As nicotine narrows your blood vessels, it will also make the insulin you have injected have more difficulty in circulating to where it is needed to digest your food. This may lead to you needing higher doses of insulin, but its effects will vary so you may not know where you are.

To give you a few figures: tobacco kills four times as many people as the total killed by drink, drugs, murder, suicide, road accidents, rail accidents, air accidents, poisoning, drowning, fires, falls, snake bites, lightning and every known cause of accidental death put together EACH YEAR.

Most heavy smokers die of diseases caused by smoking, and every cigarette you smoke shortens your life expectancy by 14 minutes. If you are female, you are less likely to be able to take the contraceptive pill safely if you smoke. Also, if you smoke while you are pregnant, you may damage your baby.

If that lot isn't enough to put you off smoking, it is also very expensive and you, your clothes and your home smell foul and develop brown stains. Also, if you smoke around people who don't smoke, you are passing on the same health hazards to them. If you are interested in keeping your environment 'green', just consider how many trees get cut down to make each packet of cigarettes.

If you are unfortunately already hooked on smoking, decide now that you can and will stop smoking. There is help available in most localities if you need it — it can be easier to give up if you have support from others. Ask your GP, hospital clinic, library or Citizens Advice Bureau for contacts.

A few final words about drugs of all sorts (and that includes alcohol). Can you think of any advantages of using them? If you can, then try and think of non-harmful ways you can gain the same advantages. There are other enjoyable ways of being 'one of the crowd', relaxing and living a full life.

Chapter 17

Driving

People with insulin dependent diabetes *can* have a driving licence, but there are more forms to fill in. To start with, you must tell the Drivers and Vehicle Licensing Centre (DVLC) in Swansea that you have insulin dependent diabetes. If you already hold a driving licence, you should write and tell the Drivers Medical Branch, DVLC, Swansea SA1 1TU about developing diabetes now, immediately, or your licence won't be valid.

When applying for a provisional driving licence, you have to answer various questions about your capacity to drive, so this is where diabetes is mentioned. The details you give must include that you are treated with insulin. When you send this form in, the DVLC will then send you another form asking more detailed questions about your diabetes.

At present the form requires you to say if you have laser treatment to your eyes or if you have any loss of sensation in your hands and/or feet. There are also questions about recognizing hypoglycaemia and having hypos in general. If the question is still the same when you read this, you are likely to have to say yes to having hypos, but, providing this is true, you should add that you have not needed any outside assistance to correct this.

You will need to provide the name and address of the doctor looking after your diabetes and give your consent for the DVLC to contact your doctor direct. This is where you need to be sure you have been responsible about your diabetes in the months leading up to your licence application. If you have been admitted to hospital with severe hypo-glycaemia, the issue of your licence may be delayed until you have gone six months without a hospital admission for hypoglycaemia. In view of these various forms, you would be wise to apply for your licence some time in advance (you can apply up to three months before your seventeenth birthday), or try to accept or expect that there may be a delay.

All this does *not* mean you will be refused a licence, providing your diabetes is well balanced and you have no complications that would spoil your safety as a driver. Your licence will be issued for a maximum of three years and will be renewed free of charge. You will have to fill in the forms again with each renewal, and the forms will be sent to you automatically. (Don't forget to notify the DVLC if you change your address during the three years.)

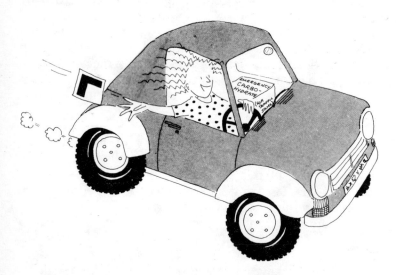

Unless the law changes, you will not be able to hold a Public Service Vehicle (PSV) licence (this means you can't drive buses) or a Heavy Goods Vehicle (HGV) licence (which means you can't drive lorries). Very rarely, if a person develops insulin dependent diabetes after they have already had one of these licences for several years, they may be able to keep it — just in case you hear of someone taking insulin who drives a bus or lorry. However, as a teenager, this is unlikely to apply to you, so you will have to accept that these licences are out for you, as are jobs that require you to have them. You can still drive vans, campers and small mini-buses, and tow trailers or caravans. There are no special restrictions for people with insulin dependent diabetes that relate to the types of motor bike you can ride.

Motor Insurance

You must tell your insurance company that you have insulin dependent diabetes — even if the questions on the proposal form don't specifically mention it. If you haven't said you have insulin dependent diabetes and you make a claim, you could find your insurance cover is null and void on the grounds of non-disclosure. If when you are learning to drive your name is added to the policy which is held by someone else, the company must again be told about your diabetes.

It pays to shop around for insurance cover as prices vary a lot and, all other things being OK, you should be able to avoid being loaded just for having diabetes. You are likely to be loaded because of your age anyway, though. You might like to try the insurance brokers that advertise in the BDA's magazine, *Balance*, and get them to do the shopping around for you.

Precautions

You should not drive if:

- you are new to diabetes — wait until your stabilization is complete
- you can't recognize the early warning signs of hypoglycaemia
- you have problems with your eyesight that can't be corrected with glasses
- you have numbness or weakness in any of your limbs.

Being hypo while driving a vehicle could be fatal, both to yourself and to other people. If you are irresponsible about this, please remember that it isn't just your licence that may go, you put at risk the licences of every other person with insulin dependent diabetes.

To avoid hypos when going on a journey, take a meal or snack no more than two hours before you drive, as a first precaution. If in doubt about your blood sugar level before leaving on a journey, do a blood test and eat something if necessary.

You must carry carbohydrate in the car (preferably both the quickly absorbed sugar and something more slowly absorbed). Ideally try to eat every two hours — though this will depend on your insulin regime. Traffic jams may make you late for a meal. Remember too that if you have to change a wheel or push the car, that takes energy, which is where you will need the extra quick-acting carbohydrate.

If you notice your hypo warning signs while driving:

- STOP immediately if it is safe to do so and don't drive on until you have eaten to raise your blood sugar.
- Remove the ignition key and leave the driving seat until your hypo symptoms have disappeared. This makes it clear that you are no longer in charge of the car/vehicle so that you cannot be accused later in court of driving while under the influence of a drug. (Insulin is classified as a drug in the eyes of the law.)

If you have an accident while hypo, you may be charged with dangerous or careless driving, or driving under the influence of a drug. Whatever the result of the charge (whether you are found innocent or guilty) your licence may be taken away. You can always appeal to the court, but you would need to be able to prove that the hypo was due to unusual circumstances and that the likelihood of the same thing happening again was remote. Even if you keep your licence, your insurance will then certainly be loaded.

If you are on a long journey, you would be wise to carry your insulin as well as food, just in case you break down and are stuck for some hours.

Finally, as with everyone else who drives, don't ever drink and drive, not even one drink.

Chapter 18

Further Education and Jobs

Exams

Exams are stressful. So what may happen to your blood sugar? Yes, it may go up.

Because you will (presumably!) be revising before an exam, you will also be having less exercise, which can be another cause of higher blood sugars. On the other hand, you may eat less if you are nervous, which may lower your blood sugar. So it is the usual personal minefield you have to negotiate.

If you can bear to, the ideal is to test your blood sugar just before you start each exam and eat if necessary. Don't inject

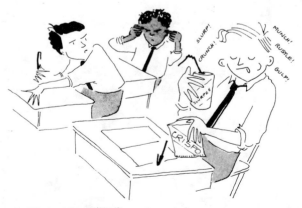

....CRISPS ARE **UNKIND** TO YOUR COLLEAGUES....

extra insulin if your blood sugar is high. This is too risky —
you might be hypo before the end of the paper, as your stress
is likely to lessen as you get into the exam. Well done if you
feel you can test your blood sugar before an exam, but try not
to worry about it if you can't — that is the 'ideal world'
solution and most of us don't live there often.

It is essential that the invigilator knows that you have
diabetes and that you may need to eat during the exam.
You must take food into the examination room, and do be
thoughtful about what you take to eat. It needs to be
something that you can unwrap and eat quietly — packets of
crisps are unkind to your colleagues!

If you should be unwell during an exam, as with anyone
else, the examining board will be notified. This will not,
however, give you a better grade. Nor will having diabetes
mean you will be allowed extra time to answer the questions.
Beware of using diabetes as an excuse during exams; it is not
a good way to make friends and influence people.

There are ways to ease the stress of exams. These will work
for people without diabetes too; their blood sugar also rises
with stress. You might like to share some of these tips with
your friends.

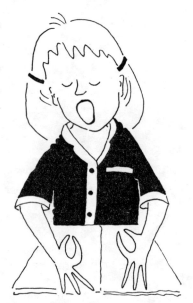

DEEP BREATHS WILL HELP....

- Try not to give up exercise totally. Even just a few short walks round the block will help to clear your head so you'll take in more and get your energy going again.
- Make yourself a timetable and take regular exercise and meal breaks.
- Spending a few minutes each day on some form of meditation will help your concentration.
- Take a few long, deep breaths before you start reading the exam question paper.

By the way, the exam stress is similar to when you take something like a driving test — certainly the deep breaths before you get into the car will help.

Very few people actually enjoy exams, but when you are looking for a job they come in handy. Having some certificates to your credit will help to show people that having diabetes doesn't mean you are incapable in any way.

College and/or further education

The fact that you have diabetes does not need to be part of your decision about going to college, university or any other sort of further education after school. Many people with diabetes have been on these types of courses before and survived.

If there is a health question on any application form, answer along the lines of 'Health good — well-controlled insulin dependent diabetic' is a way to start (assuming that it would be a true answer!) You can always add supporting letters from your diabetic clinic doctor and your teachers at school. Your teachers can show that you have good attendance records, which always helps. It is up to you to make sure your teachers can truthfully say your school attendance was good.

There is no reason why you should not go away to college or university if you would like to and have the brains to do so. If you will be living in a hall of residence, the decision about sharing a room or being on your own does not need to be made on the grounds of having diabetes. Just ask yourself which you would prefer on social grounds (and beware of parental over-protection here as well).

If you are given a local education authority grant while you are on a course, you may be able to get a little extra money because you have diabetes. (You see, sometimes 'the system' does work to your advantage!) Local authorities vary but you will lose nothing by applying for a part of the 'Disabled Students Allowance'.

You need to make a case by stating that you will need more money for food because you need to buy between-meal snacks, and possibly you will have to replace 'unsuitable' puddings if you have to eat in a hall of residence. You must give an indication of the actual costs you consider you will have to cover, and you must base this only on the number of weeks in the year you will be on your course. You may also get a little extra still on the grounds of having to buy more expensive shoes. This is always worth a try, but there are no guarantees of success.

You may find college medical staff have little detailed knowledge of diabetes, so you would be wise to get a letter from your diabetic team at home to introduce you to the one near your college — just in case you ever need them. You would be well advised to make sure the college authorities know you have diabetes, to prevent them throwing a wobbly if they find your syringes and draw the wrong conclusions about illegal drugs.

See Chapter 19 for some more points about leaving home.

Careers, jobs and employment

Let's get the down side out of the way first. There are some occupations that are barred to people with insulin dependent diabetes. At present they are:

- the armed forces and merchant navy
- the police force, fire brigade and ambulance service
- driving public service or heavy goods vehicles
- airline pilot
- deep sea diving
- mining.

You may hear of people in these jobs who have insulin dependent diabetes. If so, they will have developed diabetes *after* they started the job. Things do change so you should check the up-to-date position when you are actually on the job market. But you would be wise not to set your heart on any of these. Otherwise, you will find there are people with insulin dependent diabetes in all walks of life, all professions — and that includes many professional sports people.

To start with, you go about finding a job the same way as everyone else does. Basically, think about what you enjoy doing and talk to people about how to go about making money while doing what you enjoy. Find out as much as you can. 'People' means teachers, careers officers, friends and family.

You must tell your employer that you have diabetes. Emotionally, it won't help you if you regard diabetes as a handicap and practically, you don't want to run the risk of being fired for dishonesty. When and how you tell an employer needs thinking about.

There is no need to mention diabetes when writing or phoning for an application form. If there is a health question on the form, something like 'health good — well-controlled insulin dependent diabetic' may be the best thing to say. You can get back-up letters from your doctor and teachers. Employers will be most concerned about time off work so get your school to mention your excellent attendance record and the doctor to mention that you can attend clinics in the evening. (It's up to you to make sure that it is possible to make statements like this about you!)

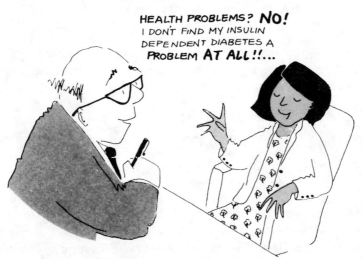

Whether or not there is a health question on a form, you would be wise to bring up diabetes in the interview. Don't assume that employers will discriminate against people with diabetes. It is, however, quite likely that they are unaware (possibly even misinformed) about the facts of diabetes. An interview is to sell yourself, and that includes selling the assets of diabetes.

People with diabetes often feel that they have to 'prove themselves' and studies show that they have an above-average work record. Living with diabetes requires a lot of self-discipline so you are likely to be a good time-keeper and generally self-aware. You will know how your body feels in relation to food and exercise. This often means that you are sensitive to other people's feelings too. Knowing what your life depends on can also give you a strength of purpose that is an asset in any job. Are you getting the idea?

Your work colleagues need to know about hypos. You can reassure them by stressing that most hypos can be prevented by eating regularly and that they are very short-lived and easily relieved within a minute or so by taking sugar. Severe hypos involving loss of consciousness are extremely rare. You can also emphasize that you have adequate warning symptoms and so will not be a danger to yourself or others. Please don't be embarrassed about eating snacks — people are rarely embarrassed by needing to light a cigarette, are they?

When you start work you may find your schedule will be quite different from the school timetable. So you may need to alter your insulin and/or food regime. Think about this beforehand, perhaps talk to your diabetic hospital team, and do more blood tests to find out where you are for a while. It will be worth it in the long run.

Registering as disabled

As someone with diabetes you are, at the time of writing, allowed to register as disabled. It is up to you to decide whether you want to do this. It may be an advantage if you live in an area of high unemployment where employers are keen to have their 3 per cent registered disabled on their workforce. (Companies over a certain size are required by law to have 3 per cent of their workforce registered as disabled.) You may also get increased access to training this way. You do not register for life, you can de-register whenever you want — something to think about.

Grey areas to be aware of:
Driving: There is no reason why you can't drive a 'company' car or van, but you will need to make sure the insurers are informed of your diabetes (see the section on driving).
Pensions: Having diabetes shouldn't bar you from a company pension plan. It is possible that your contributions will be loaded, but they needn't be. Seek advice from an appropriate expert if necessary.
Private Health Plans: These are at the moment wary of covering individuals with diabetes but you may be accepted under a company scheme. They may refuse to cover 'pre-existing conditions', which may limit your benefits considerably.

Finally, yes, you may get rejected for a job you want, and yes, it may be due to diabetes. If the firm has employed an 'unreliable' person with diabetes in the past, you may be tarred with the same brush. This is bad luck, but don't take it as a personal slight.

You may meet an employer who is prejudiced against anyone with so-called 'health problems' who will turn you down. That is their loss, it doesn't mean you are incapable. It also probably wouldn't be a very pleasant environment in which to work.

As a last resort, if you are sure you have been discriminated against solely on grounds of having diabetes, you can take legal action. However, this is very fraught and though you may get financial compensation if you win, you still won't have a job, and it may go against you when applying for other jobs. This is not really a recommended course of action.

Chapter 19

Leaving Home

It is likely that you will leave home at some point in your adult life. If you go to college or choose a job in another area, or for lots of other reasons, it may be while you are still in your teens. Even though you may be a bit nervous, this will be an exciting move for you. Don't forget though that you will be a loss for any family you leave behind. If your mother, for instance, has spent quite a time each day doing things towards your diabetes (extra food perhaps), there will be a gap for her.

If you think there might be a gap when you've moved, try to be a little understanding when you get the third phone call in a week which asks if you've taken your insulin and are you eating properly! It'll lessen with time as you show you can cope away from the 'nest'.

There are no diabetic reasons why you shouldn't live alone, share a flat or house, or take lodgings. The considerations affecting which is best for you depend on your personality, and your finances, not your diabetes. If you will feel happier if someone is around in case you go hypo in the night, by all means set this up.

When you are at the stage of buying somewhere to live, you should have no trouble getting a mortgage, providing you have some money.

If you want a mortgage with life insurance attached (an endowment mortgage rather than a straight repayment mortgage), you may find you have a loaded premium (perhaps 10 per cent) and you are likely to have to fill in forms about your diabetes and undergo a medical. Once again, companies differ, so use a broker (the BDA has one) to shop around for you.

Diabetes is no bar to long-term relationships or marriage, but do beware of dropping into a relationship because you find being responsible for your own welfare a struggle and you want someone to look after you. This isn't usually a basis for a relationship where both people grow into whole people. The ups and downs of relationships are stressful in both nice and nasty ways as you probably already know, and the downs especially are likely to mean your diabetes will be more difficult to cope with.

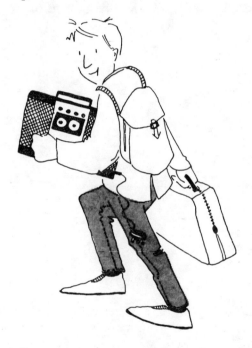

At times like these, you may find it a help to know other people with diabetes around your own age (or perhaps a bit older; they may have been through your crisis and come out the other side). Some people like to be part of a youth diabetes group, or you may prefer just to talk to one other kindred spirit. Your clinic should be able to help with contacts, as can the BDA Youth Department. If you fancy having a penfriend with diabetes, try the ads in *Balance*.

This doesn't mean to suggest that you should spend all your time associating with people with diabetes — that could lead to diabetes taking over all your life, which isn't healthy. It is sometimes good to share your feeling about diabetes with someone who has similar things to live with, though — this often helps you to cope with any downs and to get tips about how to deal with new experiences.

When you have been diagnosed for a while, you might like to offer to meet people who have been just recently diagnosed (suggest this to your diabetic team). Remembering how you felt when you were diagnosed, and sharing how you have managed, can give a lot of confidence to someone new to diabetes. Their family might be helped by talking to you and asking you questions too.

Chapter 20

Holidays and Travel

Having diabetes doesn't mean you have to restrict your holiday or travel plans. As with everything else, though, a little pre-planning makes things easier and there is some basic information you need to know.

Please don't ever feel that you must only stay in places that cater specially for people with diabetes. Wide varieties of food are available all over nowadays, and don't be put off unfamiliar dishes — you will be able to make an educated guess about the carbohydrate content. You can always compensate later by altering your insulin if necessary, if blood tests show you are out either way.

Car travel usually means (traffic jams permitting) you can stop when you like, but do make sure that you have food available in the car. Don't leave your insulin in the glove compartment or on the parcel shelf or in the boot where it might get too hot. It might be worth investing in an insulated bag or wide-necked flask for storing spare bottles while travelling.

If you get travel sick, you can take any of the pills available from a chemist to prevent this. (They may make your mouth dry. Don't get confused if this is one of your symptoms of a high blood sugar.)

Train travel means you may be subject to delay. Again, carry food and drink. Not all trains have buffet cars, and their availability is sometimes variable without notice. Not all buffet cars will have a supply of sugar-free drinks either.

Try not to feel that you *have* to disappear to the loo to inject yourself or do a blood test. Most other people don't actually notice your activities, and if they do, a few words about diabetes will be doing your bit to educate the rest of the world.

Boat travel most usually means ferries, which generally have plenty of food available. If it's a car ferry, don't leave your insulin, etc. in the car as you can't get access to your car during the voyage without a lot of palaver.

Travel abroad

If you go on a package tour, please note that the company's travel insurance is likely to exclude 'pre-existing conditions', which means diabetes in your case. Therefore, you would be wise to take out your own insurance, perhaps via the BDA's insurance brokers. If you go to Europe, EEC countries have reciprocal medical cover (get form E111 from your local DSS office to get a certificate to prove you are eligible for treatment). Even then, cover may not be as comprehensive as it is in the UK.

Wherever you go, you should take more than enough insulin, syringes and blood testing supplies with you. They may not be readily available in other countries and some European countries have insulins of different strengths. You can get enough insulin from your doctor to see you through a holiday.

If you are away for months, you will need to arrange for local supplies, which may be difficult in very out of the way places. The British Embassy might be a good contact; they might keep a parcel for you, perhaps. It can be tricky to rely on ordinary mail services as the supplies might go astray or be kept at the wrong temperature. Getting someone to act as courier might be possible, too. Don't let this put you off exotic travel; as you will read in the press, people with insulin dependent diabetes go on all sorts of expeditions — it just, as usual, needs pre-planning.

Remember about keeping your insulin reasonably cool, though insulin will remain fully active for at least one month at 25°C (77°F). You should carry some form of identification with you, and a translation of your ID card may be helpful in some places. For customs, again particularly in exotic places, a letter from your clinic explaining why you have syringes and needles is also a good idea.

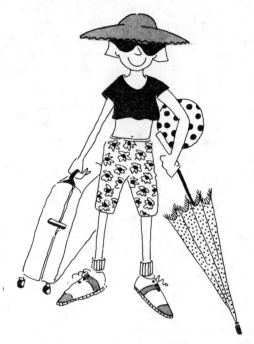

Please note that the Mark 1 Novo-pen, being metal, shows up on the metal detector at airports. You are very likely to have to take it out and explain that it is not a weapon!

You can be vaccinated against yellow fever, cholera, etc., and take the same preventive measures (for holiday tums for instance) as anyone without diabetes. Do get the vaccinations done in plenty of time before you go away, they can make you feel a bit groggy for a day or two. You would be wise also to make sure you have up-to-date cover against tetanus. (That is a good idea for anyone, travelling or not, particularly if you might be liable to sporting or driving accidents.)

You should take the same precautions to avoid tummy upsets as far as possible too. That is, beware of unbottled water (ice-cubes too): peel fruit, make sure shell-fish is fresh and well cooked. If you do get a dose of vomiting and diarrhoea, treat it as you would at home. If you can't get it sorted out in 24 hours, call a doctor. If the worst comes to the worst, the travel insurance you have taken out (you have, haven't you?!) should make it possible to fly you home.

If you feel it would be useful to know a few phrases in the appropriate language about diabetes,the BDA produces travel guides to several countries which include a useful vocabulary. If you are going somewhere that the guides don't cover, try to find someone to teach you some words of value before you go if you'll feel more confident that way. Contact your closest university or the country's embassy for help.

Air travel

Most airlines provide food very frequently, but do carry extra in case of delays. It is not usually advisable to ask for a 'diabetic' diet; you are likely to get lettuce and a piece of ham! It is worth checking that they will have sugar-free drinks on board though: soda water gets boring. Unless you are rushing about with lots of bags changing planes frequently, you may find that the lack of exercise on the flight and the excitement means your sugars are higher. This will do you no harm for the flight duration.

Vital point: always keep all your insulin and supplies with you. The hold of an aeroplane can get very cold en route which won't do insulin any good, and your baggage for Majorca may end up in Madras!

Long flights may mean you will face time-zone changes. There are various different ways of coping with this. (This is a time when it really is worth writing down what you did so you can keep track.)

Going *east*, the day is shorter. One option is to have your usual morning insulin and reduce the evening dose by 10 per cent. Going west, the day is longer and you may need an extra dose of short-acting insulin if your long-acting insulin has 'run out', plus another snack. Keep testing! On a very long flight, if you are on multiple injections, you could omit your long-acting insulin and give 2 units of short-acting each hour, plus extra for meals (it means staying awake though).

You might be wise to have two watches, or carry a clock as well. Keep one timepiece on British time until you arrive to make calculations easier. You would be well advised always to inject yourself in your seat (by which I don't mean your injection site!) It is very difficult to get to the loo when they are serving food and you never know exactly when your tray will arrive.

The BDA travel guides contain hints about local foods. You can get the address of the local diabetic association if you feel it might be helpful.

By the way, don't worry if, on a very long flight — say Britain to Australia, your ankles swell up. This is due to not moving about enough, nothing to do with diabetes. They will go down a few hours after you land. You can help prevent this by walking up and down the aisles and sitting with your feet raised if you can. Wear loose shoes too!

Above all, travel and holidays are meant to be fun, so don't make too much of a meal of diabetes or let it put you off travelling. If you fancy emigrating, uncomplicated diabetes shouldn't be a bar. Remember that health care may be different though in other countries, so sort out your options on this before you go. Australia and New Zealand have comprehensive diabetes care. In the United States you need private health insurance which can be expensive. In all countries, including the UK, care varies from area to area.

Section D

The Future

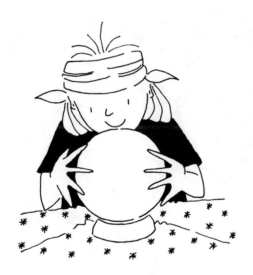

Chapter 21

Research

At the present time, there is no means of curing or preventing diabetes. So where has all the research got to, and where might it go?

With insulin dependent diabetes, we still don't understand how it is caused. In fact, we don't know how any type of diabetes is caused, unless someone has their pancreas removed by surgery — they might have cancer of the pancreas, for instance. It is difficult to examine a faulty pancreas in a living body. You have genes that give you a chance of getting diabetes but we don't know what triggered your insulin cells to destroy themselves. Perhaps a virus causes cells in your pancreas to break down and produce blood proteins ('islet cell antibodies') which continue this destructive process.

It now seems that this process of destruction is a slow process (several months or even years) so this may give time to stop the damage and stop diabetes developing in the future. The drug cyclosporin seems to slow down the destructive process, but it has very nasty side-effects so is not a 'magic' solution for now.

A few people have had pancreas transplants, but these have been people with other problems too — maybe a kidney transplant was also needed. This a long and technically difficult operation, and the number carried out in the last ten years is still only in the hundreds. Most (over 200) have been carried out in a centre in Minnesota in the USA.

Ten per cent of the people who have a pancreas transplant are dead within a year and only 50 per cent will still be insulin *in*dependent after a year. Drugs (like cyclosporin, which has nasty side-effects) need to be taken afterwards daily for the rest of your life to prevent rejection. These operations so far have only been carried out on people with advanced diabetic complications and there is little evidence to show that the pancreas transplant reverses any other complications (e.g. eye damage) that you may have. It is not known if the transplant will protect you from developing heart disease later. Also, you may again destroy these transplanted cells, so this is not yet a treatment for mass use.

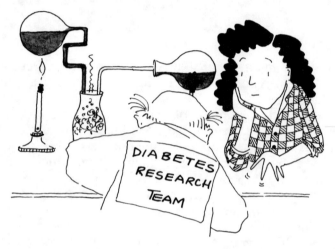

More promisingly, in the future it might be possible just to transplant insulin-producing cells, and this is being tried out in animals now. The cells are contained in a membrane when they are injected, which prevents the body seeing them as 'foreign' so there would be no need to take drugs to prevent rejection. However, the membrane acts a bit like a tea-bag and there would be problems if the holes got blocked up so the insulin could no longer be released. It will be headline news when/if it becomes possible to use this in humans, so don't worry about missing it!

Research in Japan is apparently concentrating on trying to produce an insulin 'pill' that could be taken by mouth. The problem is to find a covering for the insulin which doesn't get digested in your stomach, so that the insulin is not destroyed before it would be useful for digesting food in your gut (which is further down the tube than your stomach). In America, people are trying to develop an insulin spray that you would squirt up your nose. Nice idea, but apparently you need a lot of squirts to get much insulin absorbed into your body — and what happens if you have a cold or hay fever?

It may be found that the environment also has something to do with developing diabetes. The insulin dependent type is more common the further north you live in the world. For some reason, people who have cystic fibrosis — an inherited condition where a lot of slimy fluid (mucus) is produced in

Your future

So diabetes is for you for your lifetime. Certainly, none of us would have chosen to have it, and, to be totally honest, sometimes it is awful. When you feel it is very hard to cope with, try to find a way, or a person, to express this with. Sometimes you can explain this by it being a bit like driving a car — if you've passed your test, you know how to drive safely, but, for all sorts of reasons, sometimes you may not drive very well. So sometimes you may not 'drive' the routines of diabetes very well either. That's human, it doesn't make you 'bad' or 'stupid' — we all need a break.

On the other hand, it isn't all dreadful. You might like to try drawing a 'circle of your life' sometime. Divide it up according to how you spend a typical day, e.g. time spent sleeping, eating, alone, with others, on diabetes, on sport, etc. Do you like the balance you have? If not, what would you like to change and how will you go about this? Try keeping the circle and look back at it some time in the future.

Looking at this a different way, remember the phrase about not keeping all your eggs in one basket? (If you then drop it, you will break them all!) Try imagining you have thirty eggs and three baskets. Draw the baskets and label them, perhaps, 'Myself', 'My family', and 'School/ Work'. How many eggs go in each basket? Do you want to change this? Where does diabetes fit? You can keep eggs in the fridge for later use if you want, or have more baskets.

the lungs — are much more likely to develop diabetes (about 20 per cent). They often need insulin treatment, but don't appear to develop any complications so far. Do they have something we don't, or not have something that we do? More research is needed here.

If the trigger does turn out to be a virus, this may mean that when it is isolated people can be vaccinated against diabetes if they happen to have the genes that put them at risk. This won't be of any help to you, but it might be for your children, and anyone in future generations who is carrying the gene markers that are related to developing diabetes.

There is a lot of interesting research into diabetes treatments, causes and cures going on all over the world, and a lot of money and brain power is being spent in this field. For the moment, however, you have to accept that for you, diabetes is for life, with the insulin injections being, when you look into it, the 'best' type of treatment available at the moment.

Chapter 22

Resources

The British Diabetic Association (BDA), 10 Queen Anne Street, London, W1M 0BD (071 323 1531) produces a lot of useful information, including a bi-monthly magazine, *Balance*, which will keep you up-to-date and tell you where to get hold of things like carrying cases, and insurance brokers.

It has a Youth Department that organizes activity courses for teenagers. If you are 18 or over, you can volunteer to help

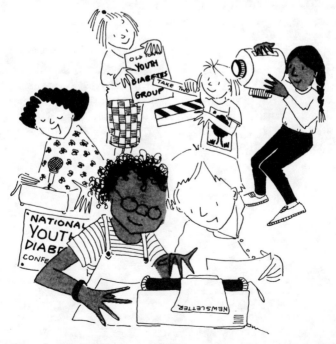

on the courses for younger children with diabetes — hard work, fun and a way to share what living with diabetes is like with others in the same boat. If your clinic or a local BDA group organizes events for people with diabetes (these may or may not be for fund-raising) you might like to help there too.

The Youth Diabetes Project, sponsored by Nordisk with the BDA, organizes a youth diabetes conference (for ages 17–25ish), a holiday course, produces a newsletter, and can help with an information pack and video if you want to start a youth diabetes group. They are at Nordisk/UK Ltd, Nordisk House, Garland Court, Garland Road, East Grinstead, West Sussex, RH19 1BR.

You can find out details of ID cards and jewellery from your clinic or the BDA.

If you need associations or people to help with other problems in your life and your family or clinic or friends won't do, try your local library, the Citizens Advice Bureau or the telephone directory.

USA and Australia

If you live in the USA, you will be able to get information and advice from the American Diabetes Association, 1660 Duke Street, Alexandria, VA 22314. Their telephone number is 703 5491500.

In Australia, contact Diabetes Australia, 149-153 Pitt Street, Redfern, NSW 2016 (02 698 1100). They can put you in touch with their offices in other states if necessary. There is also an organization specifically for young people — the Juvenile Diabetes Foundation Australia, 12/370 Victoria Avenue, Chatswood, NSW 2067 (02 411 4087). They also have offices in every state.

Afterword

And finally, for me there are people without whom this book wouldn't have been written. Those from whom I've cribbed bits of their prose, particularly Professor Jim Farquhar and Jill Pooley, thank you. Sue Bosanko for positive suggestions and the index. Graham Heys, the first person to read any of it, who, fortunately, said it was enjoyable and not boring. My best friend Simon Davey, whose 'Just get on with it!', though infuriating when I was stuck, was the most helpful and supportive thing to hear, I now admit. And, all the people, of all ages with diabetes I've listened to and shared diabetes with.

Index